OXFORD

Respiratory Problems

O G P L

OXFORD GENERAL PRACTICE LIBRARY

Respiratory Problems

Dr Jeannette Lynch

Research Fellow and General Practitioner,
University of Southampton and
Southampton, UK

and

Dr Chantal Simon

MRC Research Fellow and General Practitioner,
University of Southampton and
Christchurch, UK

and Series Editor

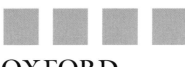

OXFORD
UNIVERSITY PRESS

OXFORD
UNIVERSITY PRESS

Great Clarendon Street, Oxford OX2 6DP

Oxford University Press is a department of the University of Oxford.
It furthers the University's objective of excellence in research, scholarship,
and education by publishing worldwide in

Oxford New York

Auckland Cape Town Dar es Salaam Hong Kong Karachi
Kuala Lumpur Madrid Melbourne Mexico City Nairobi
New Delhi Shanghai Taipei Toronto

With offices in

Argentina Austria Brazil Chile Czech Republic France Greece
Guatemala Hungary Italy Japan Poland Portugal Singapore
South Korea Switzerland Thailand Turkey Ukraine Vietnam

Oxford is a registered trade mark of Oxford University Press
in the UK and in certain other countries

Published in the United States
by Oxford University Press Inc., New York

British Library Cataloguing in Publication Data

Data available

Library of Congress Cataloging in Publication Data

Data available

Typeset by Newgen Imaging Systems (P) Ltd., Chennai, India
Printed in Italy
on acid-free paper by Legoprint S.p.A.

ISBN 978-0-19-857137-7

10 9 8 7 6 5 4 3 2 1

Contents

Acknowledgements

This book would not have come into being without the support and drive of Peter Stevenson, Dominic Stow, Emma Marchant, Sara Chare and the rest of the team at Oxford University Press.

I would also like to thank Liz Oliver for her help in reviewing this book, Dr. Francoise van Dorp for reviewing the sections relevant to paediatrics and the authors of the Women's health volume for the Oxford General Practice Library and Oxford Handbook of General Practice for allowing us to reproduce material.

All those involved in writing while working clinically, will be very aware that the real cost of such work is borne by families. I would particularly like to thank my family: Andy, Jack and Rosie, who between them have given me first-hand experience of a good proportion of the content of this book.

JL

Symbols and abbreviations

⚠	Warning
❶	Important note
🔴	Controversial point
☎	Telephone number
💾	Website
📖	Cross reference to
±	With or without
↑	Increased/increasing
↓	Decreased/decreasing
→	Leading to
1°	Primary
2°	Secondary
♂	Male
♀	Female
≈	Approximately equal
~	Approximately
%	Percent(age)
≥	Greater than or equal to
≤	Less than or equal to
>	Greater than
<	Less than
+ve	Positive
-ve	Negative
o	Degrees
£	GMS contract payment available
C	Cochrane review
G	Guideline from major guideline producing body
N	NICE guidance

R	Randomized controlled trial in major journal
S	Systematic review in major journal
ND	Notifiable disease
'	Foot/feet
"	Inches
β	Beta
AA	Attendance Allowance
AAA	Abdominal aortic aneurysm
A&E	Accident and Emergency
ACE	Angiotensin converting enzyme
AED	Automated external defibrillator
AF	Atrial fibrillation
AIDS	Acquired immuno deficiency syndrome
ALS	Advanced life support
A-V	Arterio-venous
bd	Twice daily
BCG	Bacillus Calmette-Guerin
BLS	Basic life support
BMA	British Medical Association
BMI	Body mass index
BMJ	British Medical Journal
BNF	British National Formulary
BP	Blood pressure
bpm	Beats per minute
BTS	British Thoracic Society
Ca^{2+}	Calcium
CCF	Congestive cardiac failure
CF	Cystic fibrosis
Cl^-	Chloride
cm	Centimetre(s)
CMV	Cytomegalovirus
CNS	Central nervous system
CO_2	Carbon dioxide
COC	Combined oral contraceptive

COPD	Chronic obstructive pulmonary disease
CPAP	Continuous positive airways pressure
CPR	Cardiopulmonary resuscitation
CSF	Cerebrospinal fluid
CT	Computerized tomography
CVA	Stroke
CXR	Chest X-ray
d	Day(s)
DLA	Disability Living Allowance
DM	Diabetes mellitus
DN	District nurse
DNA	Deoxyribonucleic acid
DoH	Department of Health
DTB	Drugs and Therapeutic Bulletin
DVLA	Driver and Vehicle Licensing Authority
DVT	Deep vein thrombosis
DWP	Department of Work and Pensions
EBV	Epstein-Barr virus
Echo	Echocardiogram
ECG	Electrocardiograph
e.g.	For example
ENT	Ear, nose and throat
ESR	Erythrocyte sedimentation rate
etc.	Et cetera
EU	European Union
FBC	Full blood count
FEV_1	Forced expiratory volume in one second
FH	Family history
FVC	Forced vital capacity
g	Grams
GA	General anaesthetic
GI	Gastrointestinal
GMS	General Medical Services
GORD	Gastro-oesophageal reflux disease

GP	General Practitioner
GTN	Glyceryl trinitrate
h	Hour(s)
HGV	Heavy goods vehicle
Hib	Haemophilus influenza type b
HIV	Human immunodeficiency virus
HRT	Hormone replacement therapy
ICP	Intracranial pressure
Ig	Immunoglobulin
IM	Intramuscular
INR	International normalization ratio
IS	Income support
IT	Information technology
IV	Intravenous
J	Joules
JSA	JobSeekers Allowance
JVP	Jugular venous pressure
K^+	Potassium
kg	Kilogram(s)
l	Litre(s)
L	Left
LABA	Long acting beta agonist
LMC	Local medical committee
LMWH	Low molecular weight heparin
LN	Lymph node
LRTI	Lower respiratory tract infection
LTOT	Long term oxygen therapy
LVF	Left ventricular failure
m	Metres
mcgm	Micrograms
MDI	Metred dose inhaler
mg	Milligrams
MI	Myocardial infarct
min	Minutes

ml	Millilitres
mmHg	Millimetres of mercury
mmol	Millimole
MND	Motor neurone disease
mo	Month(s)
MoD	Ministry of Defence
MRC	Medical research council
MS	Multiple sclerosis
Na^+	Sodium
NHS	National Health Service
NICE	National Institute for Clinical Excellence
NRT	Nicotine replacement therapy
NSAID	Non-steroidal anti-inflammatory drug
O_2	Oxygen
od	Once daily
OM	Otitis media
OT	Occupational theraphy/therapist
OTC	Over the counter
OUP	Oxford University Press
p.	Page number
PALS	Paediatric advanced life support
PAN	Polyarteritis nodosum
PBLS	Paediatric basic life support
PCO	Primary Care Organization
PDA	Patent ductus arteriosus
PE	Pulmonary embolus
PEFR	Peak expiratory flow rate
Physio	Physiotherapy
PMH	Past medical history
PMS	Personal Medical Services
PND	Paroxysmal nocturnal dyspnoea
po	Oral
PPI	Proton pump inhibitor
prn	As needed

PSV	Public service vehicle
qds	Four times daily
QOF	Quality and outcomes framework
R	Right
RA	Rheumatoid arthritis
RCN	Royal College of Nursing
RSV	Respiratory syncitial virus
s or sec	Second (s)
SBE	Subacute bacterial endocarditis
s/cut	Subcutaneous
SIGN	Scottish Intercollegiate Guidelines Network
SLE	Systemic lupus erythematosis
SVC	Superior vena cava
TB	Tuberculosis
tds	Three times a day
TENS	Transcutaneous electrical nerve stimulation
TFTs	Thyroid function tests
TIA	Transient ischaemic attack
TOF	Tracheo-oesophageal fistula
TV	Television
UC	Ulcerative colitis
UK	United Kingdom
URTI	Upper respiratory tract infection
UTI	Urinary tract infection
VAT	Value added tax
VF	Ventricular fibrillation
VT	Ventricular tachycardia
VZ	Varicella zoster
WCC	White cell count
wk	Week(s)
y	Year(s)

Chapter 1

Assessing patients with respiratory problems in primary care

1

Respiratory assessment

Objectives are to:
- Establish a constructive relationship with the patient to enable patient and doctor to communicate effectively, and serve as the basis for any subsequent therapeutic relationship
- Determine whether the patient has a respiratory problem and, if so, what that is
- Find out (where possible) what caused that problem
- Assess the patient's emotions and attitudes towards the problem
- Establish how it might be treated.

History: Use open questions at the start, becoming directive when necessary – clarify, reflect, facilitate, listen. *Ask about:*

Presenting complaint: Chronological account, past history of similar symptoms. Ask directly about:
- **Breathlessness (dyspnoea):** When (on exercise, during sleep – orthopnoea or PND); rate of onset; associated symptoms e.g. wheeze
- **Cough:** When (during exercise, at night); productive or dry; how long (>3wk. and no obvious cause refer for CXR^N)
- **Sputum:** Amount, colour, blood
- **Wheeze:** When (during exercise, at night, associated with URTI)
- **Pain:** Where; when; radiation; severity; duration; exacerbating/relieving factors; relationship to coughing/breathing
- **Swelling of ankles?**

Past medical history: Asthma/atopy and/or allergies; TB; heart disease; cancer

Drug history: Drugs commonly associated with respiratory problems include NSAIDs (wheeze), β-blockers (wheeze), ACE inhibitors (cough), amiodarone (pneumonitis and fibrosis), methotrexate (pulmonary fibrosis), nitrofurantoin (pulmonary fibrosis).

Social history: Smoker? Employed? Does the problem affect the job? Could the problem have been caused as a result of work? Hobbies and pets? Housing, social support etc.?

Family history: Asthma/atopy; TB; other lung disease

Attitudes and beliefs: How does the patient see the problem? What does he/she think is wrong? How does he/she think other people view the situation? What does the patient want you to do about it?

Examination: 📖 p.4

Action
- Summarize the history back to the patient and give an opportunity for the patient to fill in any gaps.
- Draw up a problem list and outline a management plan with the patient. Further investigations and interventions are guided by the findings on history and examination – so a good history and examination is essential.
- Set a review date if needed.

GP Notes: ❶ Don't forget respiratory symptoms of non-respiratory disease

- Cardiovascular disease
- Anaemia
- Depression
- Diabetes
- Thyroid disease
- Spinal dysfunction
- Anxiety and panic attacks

Figure 1.1 The respiratory assessment

Ask
Chronological history of symptoms –
- Breathlessness?
- Cough/haemoptysis?
- Sputum?
- Wheeze?
- Chest pain?
- Swelling of ankles?

Past medical history (including allergies)
Drug history
Family and social history (including smoking)

Examine
General examination – weight ↓, fever/sweats, erythema nodosum, peripheral oedema
Head and hand signs – Horner's syndrome, pallor, cyanosis, tremor, yellow nails, clubbing
Neck signs – hoarseness, stridor, lymphadenopathy, JVP, position of trachea/tracheal tug
Chest deformity – kyphosis, scoliosis, abnormal chest shape
Breathing pattern and rate
Chest signs – expansion, vocal fremitus/resonance, percussion breath sounds and added sounds

Test *Consider:*
BP, temperature
Lung function tests – peak flow and/or spirometry
Oxygen saturation
Blood – FBC and/or ESR; viral titres
Sputum culture
CXR

General examination

General inspection: Watch the patient throughout the consultation:
- How did he walk into the room? Was he breathless on exertion?
- What does the patient look like – unkempt (poor sleeper e.g. TB)? Cachectic (end-stage COPD, lung cancer, advanced heart failure)?
- Does the patient appear breathless whilst talking? Is he coughing?
- Is he in obvious discomfort or distress?
- Check temperature, BP and pulse.

Weight loss: Non-specific symptom or sign. *Consider:*
- *GI causes:* Malabsorption, malnutrition, dieting
- *Chronic disease:* Hyperthyroidism, DM, COPD, heart failure, renal disease, degenerative neurological/muscle disease, chronic infection (e.g. TB, HIV)
- *Malignancy*
- *Psychiatric causes:* Depression, dementia, anorexia.

⚠ Refer any patient with unexplained weight loss for urgent CXR[N].

Night sweats: *Consider:* TB; lymphoma; leukaemia; solid tumour (e.g. renal carcinoma); menopause; anxiety states.

Erythema nodosum: Painful, red, raised areas primarily on the shins (Figure 1.2). *Causes:*

- Infection – TB, Streptococcal, systemic fungal infection
- Drugs – sulphonamides, COC pill
- Pregnancy
- Sarcoidosis
- Inflammatory bowel disease

Peripheral oedema: Swelling of the ankles/legs (or sacrum if bed-bound) occurs when the rate of capillary filtration > rate drainage.

Is swelling acute/chronic, symmetrical/asymmetrical, localized/generalized? Are there any associated symptoms e.g. breathlessness? Treat according to cause. *Causes:*

Acute:
- DVT
- Superficial thrombophlebitis
- Cellulitis
- Joint effusion/haemarthrosis
- Haematoma
- Baker's cyst
- Arthritis
- Fracture
- Acute arterial ischaemia
- Dermatitis

Chronic:
- Gravitational oedema e.g. due to immobility – elevate feet above waist level, avoid standing still, supply support stockings (ideally apply stockings before getting out of bed). Diuretics are not a long-term solution
- Heart failure
- Venous disease – post-thrombotic syndrome, chronic venous insufficiency/venous obstruction, lipodermatosclerosis
- Hypoproteinaemia e.g. nephrotic syndrome
- Lymphoedema – infection, tumour, trauma
- Reflex sympathetic dystrophy
- Congenital vascular abnormalities

GP Notes: When assessing respiratory disease, ask yourself

Is there any evidence of respiratory distress?

- *Dyspnoea* (📖 p.22).
- *Tachypnoea:* Rapid breathing (📖 p.14).
- *Use of accessory muscles of respiration:* Patients in respiratory distress due to airways obstruction often brace the shoulder girdle by resting forwards on straight arms and using the accessory muscles of respiration (sternocleidomastoid, platysma and the strap muscles of the neck) ± abdominal muscles.
- *Nasal flaring:* A sign of respiratory distress in neonates/infants.
- *Intercostal, subcostal and/or sternal recession:* Negative intra-thoracic pressures cause indrawing of the chest wall. A sign of respiratory distress in neonates, infants and young children.
- *Wheezing* (📖 p.16) or *stridor* (📖 p.10).

Are there any signs of respiratory failure?

- ↓ level of consciousness
- Central cyanosis (📖 p.6)
- Asterixis (📖 p.6)

5

Figure 1.2 Erythema nodosum

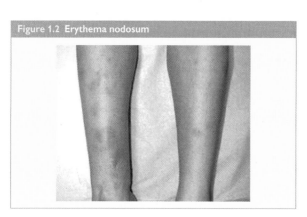

Further information

NICE Referral guidelines for suspected cancer – quick reference guide (2005) 🖥 www.nice.org.uk

Figure 1.2 is reproduced with permission from 🖥 www.studenthealth.co.uk

Head and hand signs

Horner's syndrome: Sympathetic nerve disruption to one eye results in:
- Small (meiotic) pupil with lack of pupil dilation in the dark
- Partial lid ptosis
- Anhydrosis of the forehead *and*
- Enophthalmos.

Causes
- Pancoast, cervical cord or mediastinal tumour
- Aortic aneurysm
- Posterior inferior artery or basilar artery occlusion
- Hypothalamic lesion
- Syringomyelia

Pallor: Check eyes/mucous membranes for pallor suggesting anaemia.

Cyanosis: Dusky blue skin.
Central cyanosis: Cyanosis of mucus membranes e.g. mouth. *Causes:*
- Lung disease resulting in inadequate oxygen transfer (e.g. COPD, PE, pleural effusion, severe chest infection)
- Shunting from pulmonary to systemic circulation (e.g. Fallot's tetralogy, PDA, transposition of the great arteries)
- Inadequate oxygen uptake (e.g. met- or sulf-haemoglobinaemia).

Peripheral cyanosis: e.g. cyanosis of fingers. *Causes:* as for central cyanosis plus:
- Physiological (cold, hypovolaemia)
- Local arterial disease (e.g. Raynaud's syndrome).

 Feet can be dusky blue colour due to venous disease – if this occurs without central cyanosis it does not imply abnormal oxygen saturation.

Flapping tremor/asterixis: Bilateral motor disturbance. Ask the patient to hold his hands straight out in front of him and dorsiflex his hands – this provokes a flapping, asynchronous tremor which is absent at rest. Due to CO_2 retention in severe COPD.

Yellow nails: Consider nicotine staining in chronic smokers, yellow nail syndrome (defective lymph drainage – nails grow very slowly; may be associated with pleural effusion), fungal infection, psoriasis, treatment with tetracycline.

Clubbing: Loss of the angle between nail fold and plate, bulbous finger tip and the nail fold feels boggy (Figure 1.3). *Causes:*
- *Respiratory:*
  - A – abscess, asbestosis
  - B – bronchiectasis, bronchial carcinoma (not small-cell)
  - C – cystic fibrosis, chronic infection
  - E – empyema
  - F – fibrosing alveolitis
- *Cardiac:* SBE; congenital cyanotic heart disease
- *Other:* Inflammatory bowel disease (Crohn's > UC); coeliac disease; thyrotoxicosis; biliary cirrhosis; A-V malformation; familial; idiopathic

Figure 1.3 Clubbed finger nail

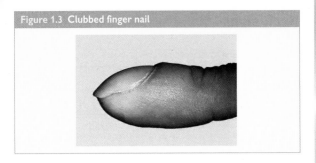

⚠ Refer any patient with unexplained nail clubbing for urgent CXR[N].

Further information
NICE Referral guidelines for suspected cancer – quick reference guide (2005) ⬚ www.nice.org.uk

Figure 1.3 is reproduced with permission from dermnet.com

Neck signs

Lymphadenopathy: Enlargement of the lymph nodes. *Causes:*
Benign:
- *Infective:*
  - Bacterial – pyogenic, TB, *Brucella*
  - Viral – EBV, CMV, HIV
  - Fungal
  - Toxoplasmosis
  - Syphilis
- *Non-infective:* Sarcoid, connective tissue disease (rheumatoid); skin disease (eczema, psoriasis); drugs (phenytoin); berylliosis

Malignant: Lymphoma, leukaemia, metastases.

Management: Refer immediately for urgent investigation if:
- Rapidly growing
- Non-tender, firm/hard lymph node >3cm diameter
- Lymph nodes associated with other unexplained signs of ill-health (night sweats, weight loss, persistent fever)
- Lymph nodes associated with other sinister signs e.g. petechial rash (same-day assessment), suspected head, neck or lung tumour
- Enlarged supraclavicular nodes in the absence of local infection.

Most enlarged lymph nodes are reactive lymph nodes – suggested by a short history, soft tender mobile lump and concurrent infection. If there are no sinister features, give these 2wk. to settle. If not settling, check FBC, ESR ± EBV screen and refer for urgent further investigation.

Hoarseness: Change in quality of the voice affecting pitch, volume or resonance. Occurs when vocal cord function is affected by a change in the cords, a neurological or muscular problem.

Causes of hoarseness:
- *Local causes:* URTI (commonest); laryngitis; trauma – shouting, coughing, vomiting, instrumentation; carcinoma; hypothyroidism; acromegaly
- *Neurological problems:* Laryngeal nerve palsy (❗ may be associated with lung cancer); motor neurone disease; myaesthenia gravis; multiple sclerosis
- *Muscular problems:* Muscular dystrophy
- *Functional problems:* Hysterical paralysis of vocal cord adductors

Assessment: Weight ↓, dysphagia or neck lumps add to suspicions of malignancy. Check TFTs in those with weight gain. Indirect laryngoscopy with a mirror can be difficult and give a poor view. ENT departments have thin fibre-optic scopes for direct visualization in outpatients.

⚠ **Refer urgently for chest X-ray (CXR)[N]:** ALL patients with hoarseness for >3wk., particularly smokers aged >50y. and heavy drinkers.

If there is a POSITIVE finding on CXR: Refer urgently to a team specializing in the management of lung cancer.

If there is a NEGATIVE finding on CXR: Refer urgently to a team specializing in the management of head and neck cancer.

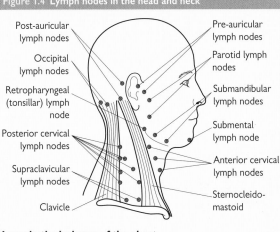

Figure 1.4 Lymph nodes in the head and neck

Post-auricular lymph nodes
Occipital lymph nodes
Retropharyngeal (tonsillar) lymph node
Posterior cervical lymph nodes
Supraclavicular lymph nodes
Clavicle

Pre-auricular lymph nodes
Parotid lymph nodes
Submandibular lymph nodes
Submental lymph node
Anterior cervical lymph nodes
Sternocleido-mastoid

Lymphatic drainage of the chest

- Lung – cervical and supraclavicular nodes (via hilum and paratracheal nodes).
- Chest wall – axillary nodes.

⚠
- Refer any patient with supraclavicular or cervical lymphadenopathy persisting >3wk. for urgent CXR[N].
- Refer any unexplained lump in the neck of recent onset, or any previously undiagnosed neck lump that has changed over a period of 3–6wk. for urgent further investigation[N].

Further information

NICE Referral guidelines for suspected cancer – quick reference guide (2005) ⊞ www.nice.org.uk

Stridor: Noise created on inspiration due to narrowing of the larynx or trachea. Much more common in children than adults.

⚠ **Signs of severe airway narrowing**
- Distress
- ↑ respiratory rate
- Pallor and cyanosis
- Use of accessory muscles and tracheal tug

Refer any patient with signs of severe airway narrowing and all adults with stridor[N] for immediate hospital assessment.

Causes:
- Congenital abnormalities of the larynx
- Epiglottitis
- Croup (laryngotracheobronchitis)
- Swelling of the trachea e.g. as a result of anaphylaxis
- Inhaled foreign body or other obstruction
- Trauma
- Laryngeal paralysis

Jugular venous pressure: Observe internal jugular vein at 45° with head turned slightly to the left. Vertical height is measured in relation to the sternal angle. Raised if >4cm.

Causes of ↑ JVP:
- Fluid overload
- Right heart failure and CCF
- SVC obstruction (non-pulsatile)
- Tricuspid or pulmonary valve disease
- Pulmonary hypertension
- Arrhythmia – AF or atrial flutter, complete heart block
- ↑ intrathoracic pressure e.g. pneumothorax, PE, emphysema

The trachea: Figure 1.5
- Palpate the trachea in the supraclavicular notch in the midline.
- Deviation to the left or right suggests a shift of the upper mediastinum to that side.
- The distance between the suprasternal notch and cricoid cartilage in an adult is 2–3 finger breadths. If it is less than this, the lungs are probably hyperinflated.

Further information

NICE Referral guidelines for suspected cancer – quick reference guide (2005) ▣ www.nice.org.uk

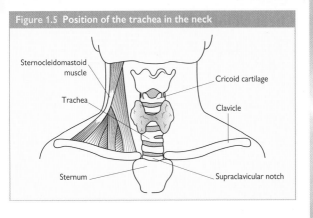

Figure 1.5 Position of the trachea in the neck

Chest deformity

Barrel chest: (Figure 1.6b) The antero-posterior diameter of the chest is high compared to the lateral diameter, and expansion is ↓. Ribs move in a pump handle, up-and-down motion. Associated with chronic hyperinflation (e.g. asthma or COPD).

Pigeon chest (pectus carinatum): (Figure 1.7) Prominent sternum and flat chest associated with history of chronic childhood asthma or rickets.

Funnel chest (pectus excavatum): (Figure 1.8) The lower end of the sternum is depressed. Often inherited or idiopathic and usually harmless.

Kyphosis: (Figure 1.9) ↑ forward spinal convexity. Usually affects the thoracic spine.
- *Postural kyphosis* ('drooping shoulders' or 'roundback') is common and voluntarily correctable.
- *Structural kyphosis* cannot be corrected voluntarily. *Common causes:* osteoporosis, Paget's disease, ankylosing spondylitis, and adolescent kyphosis – Scheuermann's disease. May cause a restrictive ventilatory defect and eventually lead to respiratory failure.

Scoliosis: (Figure 1.10) ↑ lateral curvature of the spine. Above and below the scoliosis, secondary curves develop to maintain normal position of head and pelvis. In all cases refer to orthopaedics for assessment.
- *Non-structural scoliosis* ('mobile scoliosis') is usually secondary to an abnormality outside the spine e.g. unequal leg length. It disappears when that is corrected.
- *Structural scoliosis* ('true scoliosis') is non-correctable. *Causes:* idiopathic, neuromuscular (e.g. cerebral palsy, muscular dystrophy, neurofibromatosis), trauma, osteoporosis, TB of the spine (rare), spinal tumours (rare), congenital abnormalities of the spine (rare). Can eventually cause respiratory failure.

Harrison's sulcus: Groove deformity of the lower ribs at the diaphragm attachment site. Suggests chronic childhood asthma or rickets.

Scars: Are there any scars indicative of previous chest surgery?

Surgical emphysema: Air in the subcutaneous tissue. Can be caused by spontaneous pneumothorax or trauma to the chest wall. Tissues appear swollen and crackle on palpation.

Figure 1.6 (a) Normal and (b) Barrel chest

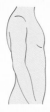

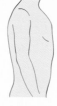

Cross-section

(a)   (b)

Reproduced with permission from Lippincott, Williams & Wilkins. Instructor's resource CD-ROM to accompany *Fundamentals of Nursing: the art and science of nursing care* (5th edn).

Figure 1.7 Pigeon chest

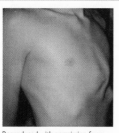

Reproduced with permission from www.answers.com

Figure 1.8 Funnel chest

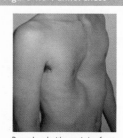

Reproduced with permission from www.answers.com

Figure 1.9 Kyphosis

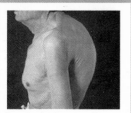

Reproduced with permission from www.megru.unizh.ch/j3/innere/pneumologie/copd05.html

Figure 1.10 Scoliosis

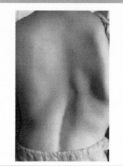

Breathing rate and pattern

Respiratory rate: Normal rate for an adult is 14 breaths/min. at rest. Higher in children:

- Neonate: 30–60 breaths/min.
- Infant: 20–40 breaths/min.
- 1–3y.: 20–30 breaths/min.
- 4–10y.: 15–25 breaths/min.
- >10y.: 15–20 breaths/min.

↑ respiratory rate: Consider:
- Lung disease e.g. pneumonia, asthma
- Heart disease e.g. LVF
- Metabolic disease e.g. ketoacidosis
- Drugs e.g. salicylate overdose
- Psychiatric causes e.g. hyperventilation.

↓ respiratory rate: Consider:
- CNS disease e.g. CVA
- Drugs e.g. opiates.

Cheyne-Stokes respiration: Breathing becomes progressively deeper and then shallower (±episodic apnoea) in cycles. *Causes:* brainstem lesions/compression (stroke, ↑ ICP); chronic pulmonary oedema; poor cardiac output. It is enhanced by narcotics.

Hyperventilation: May be fast (>20 breaths/min.) or deep (tidal volume ↑). If inappropriate results in palpitations, dizziness, faintness, tinnitus, chest pains, perioral and peripheral tingling (due to plasma Ca^{2+} ↓).

Causes include:
- Anxiety (commonest cause)
- PE
- Early pulmonary oedema
- Hyperthyroidism
- Fever
- Lymphangitis
- Weakness of the respiratory muscles.

Kussmaul respiration: Deep, sighing breathing that is principally seen in metabolic acidosis e.g. diabetic ketoacidosis and uraemia.

Neurogenic hyperventilation: Hyperventilation produced by stroke, tumour or CNS infection.

Hypoventilation: Abnormally decreased pulmonary ventilation. Respiration may be too slow or tidal volume ↓. *Causes include:*
- Respiratory depression e.g. opiate analgesia, anoxia, trauma
- Neurological disease e.g. Guillain-Barré Syndrome, polio, motor neurone disease, syringobulbia
- Lung disease e.g. pneumonia, collapse, pneumothorax, pleural effusion
- Respiratory muscle disease e.g. myasthenia gravis, dermatomyositis
- Limited chest movement e.g. kyphoscoliosis.

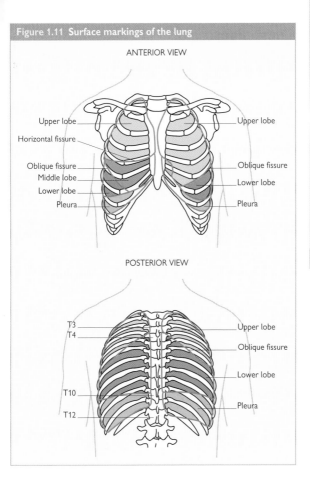

Figure 1.11 Surface markings of the lung

Chest signs

Chest expansion: Place a hand on each side of the chest over the upper then lower zones. Watch the movement of the hands during respiration - movement should be symmetrical and equal. If not suspect chest pathology (e.g. consolidation, collapse, pneumothorax, effusion) on the side with decreased movement

Vocal Fremitus/resonance: Place a hand or stethoscope on the chest wall at intervals over the chest wall (as in Figure 1.12), and ask the patient to say '99'. In the normal chest, through the stethoscope, sound is slightly unclear. Some vibrations can be felt on the chest wall.

- ↑ *transmission* implies consolidation. Even whispered sounds are heard clearly with a stethoscope (**whispering pectoriloquy**).
- ↓ *transmission* implies something in the way blocking the transmission of sound. *Consider:* air (e.g. pneumothorax), fluid (e.g. effusion), pleural thickening.

Percussion: For a right handed examiner (reverse if left handed) place the middle finger of the left hand firmly against the chest wall, lifting the palm and other fingers clear of the chest wall. Sharply tap the middle phalanx of the left middle finger with the tip of the middle finger of the right hand. Repeat at intervals over the anterior, posterior and lateral chest wall as in Figure 1.12 comparing left side with right. Define any areas of dullness to percussion by percussing from a resonant to dull area.

Interpretation:
- ↑ resonance - emphysema or pneumothorax
- ↓ resonance - consolidation, collapse, abscess, tumour, fibrosis
- Stony dullness - pleural effusion

Breath sounds: Assess character of breath sounds and added sounds:
- *Bronchial breathing:* Breath sounds are harsher than normal and there is an audible gap between inspiration and expiration - often caused by lung consolidation e.g. due to pneumonia
- ↓ *breath sounds: Consider:* pleural effusion, pneumothorax, emphysema, lung collapse
- *Added sounds:* Pleural rub; wheeze; crepitations/crackles

Pleural rub: Creaking sound produced by movement of visceral over parietal pleura when both are inflamed (e.g. pneumonia, infarction).

Wheeze: Musical sound heard during expiration.
- *Polyphonic wheeze:* indicates narrowing of many small airways - typical of asthma or COPD.
- *Monophonic wheeze:* indicates single large airway obstruction e.g. due to foreign body or tumour.

Crackles in the chest: Produced by air flow moving secretions.
- *Fine crackles:* Consider pulmonary oedema (early inspiratory – usually best heard at the lung bases at the back); early pneumonia; fibrosing alveolitis (late inspiratory).
- *Coarse crackles:* Consider TB; resolving pneumonia; bronchiectasis; lung abscess.

Figure 1.12 Systematic sequence of examination of the chest. Use the same pattern for palpation, percussion and auscultation

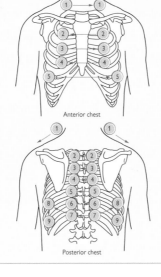

Anterior chest

Posterior chest

Table 1.1 Chest signs associated with common chest pathology

	Consolidation e.g. pneumonia	Pleural effusion	Collapsed lung	Pneumothorax
Mediastinum	Not displaced	Normal or displaced away from the effusion	Displaced towards the side of collapse	Displaced away from the side of pneumothorax
Expansion	↓	↓	↓	↓
Percussion	Dull	Stony dull	Dull	Hyper-resonant
Breath sounds	Bronchial breathing	↓	↓	↓
Added sounds	Crackles ± rub	Bronchial breathing above the effusion	None	None
Other	↑ vocal resonance, whispering pectoriloquy	↓ vocal resonance		↓ vocal resonance

⚠ Refer all patients with unexplained chest signs lasting >3wk. for urgent CXR[N].

Figure 1.12 is reproduced with permission from Lippincott, Williams & Wilkins. Instructor's resource CD-ROM to accompany *Fundamentals of Nursing: the art and science of nursing care*, (5th edn).

Chest pain

Chest pain is a common symptom.

⚠ Always think – could this be an MI, PE, dissecting aneurysm or pericariditis?

On receiving the call for assistance: *Ask:*
- Nature and location of the pain
- Duration of the pain
- Other associated symptoms – sweating, nausea, shortness of breath, palpitations
- Past medical history (particularly heart disease, high cholesterol)
- Family history (particularly heart disease)
- Smoker?

Action
- Consider differential diagnosis (Table 1.2).
- If MI is suspected call for ambulance assistance before (or instead of) visiting.
- Otherwise visit (or arrange surgery appointment), assess and treat according to cause.

Further assessment

History: Ask about:
- Site and nature of pain. Any history of trauma?
- Duration
- Associated symptoms (e.g. breathlessness, nausea)
- Provoking and relieving factors
- PMH, FH (e.g. heart disease), drug history, smoking history.

Examination:
- Check BP in both arms
- General appearance – distress, sweating, pallor
- JVP and carotid pulse
- Respiratory rate
- Apex beat
- Heart sounds
- Lung fields
- Local tenderness
- Pain on movement of chest
- Skin rashes
- Swelling or tenderness of legs (?DVT)

Investigations: ECG and CXR may be helpful.

⚠ Refer any patient with unexplained chest/shoulder pain of >3wk. duration for urgent CXR[N].

Further information
NICE Referral guidelines for suspected cancer – quick reference guide (2005) ◨ www.nice.org.uk

GP Notes:

⚠ If a patient is acutely unwell with chest pain and the cause is not clear, err on the side of caution and admit for further assessment.

19

Table 1.2 Causes of acute chest pain

Diagnosis	Features
MI	Band-like chest pain around the chest or central chest pressure/dull ache ± radiation to shoulders, arms (L>R), neck and/or jaw. Often associated with nausea, sweating and/or shortness of breath.
Unstable angina	As for MI.
Pericarditis	Sharp, constant sternal pain relieved by sitting forwards. May radiate to left shoulder ± arm or into the abdomen. Worse lying on the left side and on inspiration, swallowing and coughing.
Dissecting thoracic aneurysm	Typically presents with sudden tearing chest pain radiating to the back. Consider in any patient with chest pain (especially if radiates through to the back) and ↓BP.
PE	Acute dyspnoea, sharp chest pain (worse on inspiration), haemoptysis and/or syncope. Tachycardic and mild pyrexia.
Pleurisy	Sharp, localized chest pain, worse on inspiration. May be associated with symptoms and signs of a chest infection.
Pneumothorax	Sudden onset of pleuritic chest pain or ↑ breathlessness ± pallor and tachycardia.
Oesophageal spasm, oesophagitis	Central chest pain. May be associated with acid reflux (though not always). May be described as burning but often indistinguishable from cardiac pain. May respond to antacids.
Musculoskeletal pain	Localized pain – worse on movement. May be a history of injury.
Shingles	Intense, often sharp, unilateral pain. Responds poorly to analgesia. May be present several days before rash appears.
Costochondritis	Inflammation of the costochondral junctions – tenderness over the costochondral junction and pain in the affected area on springing the chest wall.
Bornholm's disease	Unilateral chest and/or abdominal pain, rhinitis. Coxsackie virus infection. Treat with simple analgesia.
Idiopathic chest pain	No cause apparent. Common. Affects young people > elderly people. ♀ > ♂

Cough and haemoptysis

Cough: Reaction to irritation anywhere from pharynx to lungs.

Acute cough (<3wk.): Causes:

- URTI
- Croup
- Tracheitis
- LRTI
- Pneumonia – productive, loose cough
- Acute exacerbation of asthma normally well controlled
- Inhaled foreign body – especially in well children

Reserve CXR for patients with marked focal chest signs or where inhalation of foreign body is suspected.

Management: Treat the cause where possible; advise OTC cough mixture as needed e.g. simple linctus; steam inhalation often eases symptoms temporarily; review if not clearing.

Chronic cough (>3wk.): Causes:

- Postnasal drip
- Post viral
- COPD
- Asthma
- Lung cancer
- Pertussis
- TB
- Bronchiectasis
- Pulmonary oedema
- Foreign body
- Vocal cord palsy
- GORD
- LVF
- Drug-induced (e.g. ACE inhibitors)
- Smoker's cough
- Psychogenic
- Idiopathic
- Ear wax

⚠ **Red flags:** weight ↓, night sweats.

Management: Refer any patient with a persistent cough for >3wk. for urgent CXR[N]. Treat the cause. If no cause is found, refer.

Table 1.3 Cough associations

Nocturnal	Waking	Food	Breathlessness
Asthma	Bronchiectasis	Hiatus hernia	Asthma
LVF	Chronic bronchitis	Oesophageal diverticulum	LVF
Postnasal drip	Reflux	Tracheo-oesophageal fistula	COPD
Chronic bronchitis			
Whooping cough			

Sputum

- Smoking is the leading cause of excess sputum production – look for black specks of inhaled carbon.
- Yellow–green sputum is due to cell debris (bronchial epithelium, neutrophils, eosinophils) and is not always infected.
- Bronchiectasis causes copious greenish sputum.
- Blood-stained sputum (haemoptysis) always needs full investigation. Pink froth suggests pulmonary oedema.
- Absolutely clear sputum is probably saliva.

Haemoptysis: Expectoration of blood/blood-stained sputum. *Causes:*

- Infection – bronchitis, pneumonia, lung abscess, TB
- Violent coughing
- Bronchiectasis
- Lung cancer
- PE (blood is not mixed with sputum)
- Inhaled foreign body
- Iatrogenic – anticoagulation, endotracheal tube
- Trauma
- Cardiac – acute LVF, mitral stenosis
- Blood dyscrasia/bleeding diathesis
- Idiopathic pulmonary haemosiderosis
- Bronchial adenoma
- Mycosis e.g. aspergilloma
- Goodpasture's syndrome
- Collagen vascular disease e.g. PAN, Wegener's granulomatosis
- Unknown

🛈 Differentiate from haematemesis or local bleeding from the nasopharynx or sinuses. Melaena may occur if enough blood is swallowed.

Management: Haemoptysis rarely needs treating in its own right but *always* requires investigation to find the cause.

- Admit as an acute medical emergency if the patient is compromised by the bleeding (i.e. problems with airway, tachycardia, low BP, postural drop) or has symptoms/signs of an underlying cause requiring acute admission (e.g. PE, acute LVF).
- If not compromised by the bleeding, refer for urgent CXR[N].
- Refer for urgent assessment by a chest physician if abnormal CXR, persistent haemoptysis with normal CXR in a patient aged >40y. who smokes or used to smoke, or if normal CXR but high suspicion of lung cancer[N].

🛈 In patients with lung cancer who have a massive haemoptysis, consider whether it is a terminal event. If so, consider treating with IV morphine/diamorphine and a sedative (e.g. midazolam or rectal diazepam) rather than admitting.

Further information

NICE Referral guidelines for suspected cancer – quick reference guide (2005) www.nice.org.uk

Breathlessness

Dyspnoea: Sensation of shortness of breath. Speed of onset helps diagnosis (Table 1.4). Try to quantify exercise tolerance (e.g. dressing, distance walked, climbing stairs).

> **Acute breathlessness:** Attend as soon as possible after receiving the call for help. If there is likely to be any delay, call for emergency ambulance assistance.
>
> ## On arrival
> - Be calm and reassuring. Breathlessness is frightening and panic only adds to the sensation of being breathless.
> - Direct history and examination to finding the cause as quickly as possible (Table 2.2). Treat according to the cause.
> - If no cause can be found – don't delay – admit to hospital as an acute medical emergency.

Exertional dyspnoea: Breathlessness with exercise. Causes are the same as dyspnoea generally. The New York Heart Association classifies 4 grades of severity:
- *Normal*
- *Moderate:* Walking on the level causes breathlessness
- *Severe:* Has to stop due to breathlessness when walking on the flat. All but the lightest housework is impossible
- *Gross:* Slightest effort → severe breathlessness. The patient is almost bed/chair bound.

Orthopnoea: Dyspnoea on lying flat and relieved by sitting up. Associated with left heart dysfunction e.g. LVF.

Paroxysmal nocturnal dyspnoea: Acute form of dyspnoea that causes the patient to awake from sleep. The patient is forced to sit upright or stand out of bed for relief. Associated with pulmonary oedema.

Combined chest pain and dyspnoea: *Consider:*
- MI
- Pericarditis
- Dissecting aneurysm
- PE
- Oesophageal pain
- Musculoskeletal pain
- Chest infection
- Pulmonary malignancy e.g. mesothelioma, lung cancer.

> ⚠
> - Refer any patient with symptoms/signs of superior vena cava obstruction (acute breathlessness, headache worse on stooping, swelling of the face and/or neck with fixed elevation of jugular venous pressure) for immediate medical or oncology assessment[N].
> - Refer any patient with unexplained dyspnoea of >3wk. duration for urgent CXR[N].

Table 1.4 Causes of dyspnoea

Cause	Acute	Subacute	Chronic
Cardiac disease	Acute LVF Arrhythmia Air hunger due to shock e.g. 2° to MI, dissecting thoracic aneurysm Pericarditis	Arryhthmia SBE	CCF Mitral stenosis Aortic stenosis Congenital heart disease
Lung disease	Pneumothorax Acute asthma attack PE Acute pneumonitis e.g. due to inhaling toxic gas	Asthma Infective Exacerbation of COPD Pleural effusion Pneumonia	COPD Cystic fibrosis Fibrosing alveolitis Occupational lung diseases Mesothelioma Lung cancer
Other	Hyperventilation Foreign body inhalation Guillain-Barré syndrome Altitude sickness Ketoacidosis Polio Musculoskeletal chest pain Oesophageal pain	Aspirin poisoning Myaesthenia gravis Thyrotoxicosis	Kyphoscoliosis Anaemia MND MS

Further information

NICE Referral guidelines for suspected cancer – quick reference guide (2005) ▣ www.nice.org.uk

Investigations

Indications for urgent CXR[N]
- Haemoptysis
- Any of the following if unexplained or present for >3wk.:
  - Cough
  - Chest/shoulder pain
  - Dyspnoea
  - Weight loss
  - Chest signs
  - Hoarseness
  - Finger clubbing
  - Cervical/supraclavicular lymphadenopathy
  - Signs suggesting metastases (brain, bone, liver, skin)

Peak flow: A simple and cheap test. Peak flow is not a good measure of airflow limitation as it tends to overestimate lung function. It is best used to monitor progress of disease and effects of treatment for patients with asthma. Link with self-management plan. Peak flow meters are available on NHS prescription. Peak flow charts are available from NHS supplies (form FP1010) and drug companies.

ⓘ Peak flow meters and charts changed to EU scale in 2004. Ensure both charts and meters are compatible.

Measuring peak expiratory flow rate (PEFR):
- Ask the patient to stand up (if possible) and hold the peak flow meter, horizontally. Check the indicator is at zero and the track clear.
- Ask the patient to take a deep breath and blow out forcefully into the peak flow meter, ensuring lips are sealed firmly around the mouthpiece.
- Read the PEFR off the meter. The best of 3 attempts is recorded.
- Consider using a low-range meter if predicted or best PEFR is <250l/min.
- Normal values – Table 1.5.

Interpretation of peak flow (asthma):
- 50–80% predicted or best = moderate exacerbation
- 33–50% predicted or best = severe exacerbation
- <33% predicted or best = life-threatening asthma

GP Notes:

PEFR is a relative measure only. For accurate interpretation, previous normal values for that patient are needed. Always interpret in the context of symptoms and signs.

Further information
NICE Referral guidelines for suspected cancer – quick reference guide (2005) ▣ www.nice.org.uk

Table 1.5 Predicted PEFR measurements in l/min. (EU scale)

Children: Height is the only determinant of PEFR in children. With increasing age the pattern of adult values takes over.

Height: ft	3'		3'4"	3'8"	4'	4'4"	4'8"	5'	5'4"	5'8"	6'
m	90cm		1	1.1	1.2	1.3	1.4	1.5	1.6	1.7	1.8
PEFR l/min.	88		105	136	172	220	265	313	371	427	487

Women:
Height: →

ft	4'10"	4'11"	5'	5'1"	5'2"	5'3"	5'4"	5'5"	5'6"	5'7"	5'8"	5'9"	5'10"
m	1.47	1.5	1.52	1.55	1.57	1.6	1.62	1.65	1.67	1.7	1.72	1.75	1.77
Age													
15y.	379	382	385	389	391	394	397	400	402	405	407	411	413
20y.	402	406	409	413	416	419	422	425	428	431	434	437	439
25y.	415	419	422	426	429	433	435	439	441	445	447	451	453
30y.	419	424	427	431	433	437	440	444	446	450	452	456	458
35y.	418	423	425	430	432	436	439	443	445	449	451	454	457
40y.	413	417	420	424	427	431	433	437	439	443	445	449	451
45y.	405	409	412	416	418	422	425	428	431	434	436	440	442
50y.	394	399	401	405	407	411	414	417	419	423	425	428	430
55y.	383	387	389	393	395	399	401	404	407	410	412	415	417
60y.	370	373	376	379	382	385	387	391	393	396	398	401	403
65y.	356	360	362	366	368	371	373	376	378	381	383	386	388
70y.	343	346	348	351	353	356	358	361	363	366	368	371	372

Men:
Height: →

ft	5'2"	5'3"	5'4"	5'5"	5'6"	5'7"	5'8"	5'9"	5'10"	5'11"	6'	6'1"	6'2"
m	1.57	1.6	1.62	1.65	1.67	1.7	1.72	1.75	1.77	1.8	1.82	1.85	1.87
Age													
15y.	479	485	489	494	498	503	506	511	515	520	523	528	531
20y.	534	540	545	551	555	561	565	571	575	580	584	589	593
25y.	568	575	580	587	591	598	602	608	612	618	622	628	632
30y.	587	594	599	606	611	617	622	628	633	639	643	649	653
35y.	594	601	606	613	618	625	629	636	640	646	650	657	661
40y.	592	599	604	611	615	622	627	633	637	644	648	654	658
45y.	582	590	594	601	606	612	617	623	627	634	638	644	647
50y.	568	575	580	586	591	597	601	608	612	618	622	627	631
55y.	550	557	561	568	572	578	582	588	592	598	602	607	611
60y.	529	536	540	546	550	556	560	566	570	575	579	584	588
65y.	507	513	517	523	527	533	536	542	545	551	554	559	562
70y.	484	490	493	499	503	508	511	517	520	525	528	533	536

ⓘ For normal values in age groups/heights not represented on these charts or for conversion from the old Wright scale peak flow meters see 🖥 www.peakflow.com

PEFR charts adapted from Gregg & Nunn, *BMJ* (1989) **298**: 1068–70 and Godfrey et al., *Br. J. Dis. Chest* (1970) **64**: 15.

Spirometry: Measures the volume of air the patient is able to expel from the lungs after a maximal inspiration.
- **FEV_1:** Volume of air the patient is able to exhale in the first second of forced expiration.
- **FVC:** Total volume of air the patient can forcibly exhale in 1 breath.
- **FEV_1/FVC:** Ratio of FEV_1 to FVC expressed as a %.

Measuring FEV_1 and FVC:
- Sit the patient comfortably.
- Ask the patient to take a deep breath in.
- Ask the patient to blow the whole breath out as hard as possible until there is no breath left to expel and ensuring lips are sealed firmly around the mouthpiece.
- Encourage the patient to keep breathing out.
- Repeat the procedure x 2 (i.e. 3 attempts in all).
- At least 2 readings should be within 100ml or 5% of each other.
- Normal values – Table 1.7.

Flow volume measurement: Available with some spirometers. Shape of the flow–volume curve may suggest an obstructive picture – Figure 1.13.

Table 1.6 Interpretation of spirometry results		
	Restrictive lung disease e.g. fibrosing alveolitis	**Obstructive lung disease e.g. COPD**
FEV_1 (% of predicted normal)	↓ (<80%)	↓ (<80%)
FVC (% of predicted normal)	↓ (<80%)	Normal or ↓
FEV_1/FVC	Normal (>70%)	↓ (<70%)

🛈 There may be a mixed picture.

Figure 1.13 Schematic maximum expiratory and inspiratory flow–volume curves

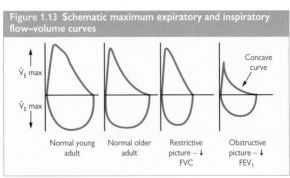

Spirometry normal values are reproduced with permission from the British Thoracic Society.

Table 1.7 Predicted FEV₁ and FVC measurements (in l)

ℹ These values apply for Caucasians. ↓ values by 7% for Asians and 13% for people of Afro-Caribbean origin.

Women:

Height	ft	4'11"	5'1"	5'3"	5'5"	5'7"	5'9"	5'11"
	m	1.5	1.55	1.6	1.65	1.7	1.75	1.8
Age								
38–41y.	FEV₁	2.3	2.5	2.7	2.89	3.09	3.29	3.49
	FVC	2.69	2.91	3.13	3.35	3.58	3.80	4.02
42–45y.	FEV₁	2.2	2.4	2.6	2.79	2.99	3.19	3.39
	FVC	2.59	2.81	3.03	3.25	3.47	3.69	3.91
46–49y.	FEV₁	2.1	2.3	2.5	2.69	2.89	3.09	3.29
	FVC	2.48	2.7	2.92	3.15	3.37	3.59	3.81
50–53y.	FEV₁	2	2.2	2.4	2.59	2.79	2.99	3.19
	FVC	2.38	2.6	2.82	3.04	3.26	3.48	3.71
54–57y.	FEV₁	1.9	2.1	2.3	2.49	2.69	2.89	3.09
	FVC	2.27	2.49	2.72	2.94	3.16	3.38	3.6
58–61y.	FEV₁	1.8	2	2.2	2.39	2.59	2.79	2.99
	FVC	2.17	2.39	2.61	2.83	3.06	3.28	3.5
62–65y.	FEV₁	1.7	1.9	2.1	2.29	2.49	2.69	2.89
	FVC	2.07	2.29	2.51	2.73	2.95	3.17	3.39
66–69y.	FEV₁	1.6	1.8	2	2.19	2.39	2.59	2.79
	FVC	1.96	2.18	2.4	2.63	2.85	3.07	3.29

For women ≥70y. use the formulae:
- $FEV_1 = (0.0395 \times \text{height in m.} \times 100) - (0.025 \times \text{age in y.}) - 2.6$
- $FVC = (0.0443 \times \text{height in m.} \times 100) - (0.026 \times \text{age in y.}) - 2.89$

Men:

Height	ft	5'3"	5'5"	5'7"	5'9"	5'11"	6'1"	6'3"
	m	1.6	1.65	1.7	1.75	1.8	1.85	1.9
Age								
38–41y.	FEV₁	3.2	3.42	3.63	3.85	4.06	4.28	4.49
	FVC	3.81	4.1	4.39	4.67	4.96	5.25	5.54
42–45y.	FEV₁	3.09	3.3	3.52	3.73	3.95	4.16	4.38
	FVC	3.71	3.99	4.28	4.57	4.86	5.15	5.43
46–49y.	FEV₁	2.97	3.18	3.4	3.61	3.83	4.04	4.26
	FVC	3.6	3.89	4.18	4.47	4.75	5.04	5.33
50–53y.	FEV₁	2.85	3.07	3.28	3.5	3.71	3.93	4.14
	FVC	3.5	3.79	4.07	4.36	4.65	4.94	5.23
54–57y.	FEV₁	2.74	2.95	3.17	3.38	3.6	3.81	4.03
	FVC	3.39	3.68	3.97	4.26	4.55	4.83	5.12
58–61y.	FEV₁	2.62	2.84	3.05	3.27	3.48	3.7	3.91
	FVC	3.29	3.58	3.87	4.15	4.44	4.73	5.02
62–65y.	FEV₁	2.51	2.72	2.94	3.15	3.37	3.58	3.8
	FVC	3.19	3.47	3.76	4.05	4.34	4.63	4.91
66–69y.	FEV₁	2.39	2.6	2.82	3.03	3.25	3.46	3.68
	FVC	3.08	3.37	3.66	3.95	4.23	4.52	4.81

For men ≥70y. use the formulae:
- $FEV_1 = (0.043 \times \text{height in m.} \times 100) - (0.029 \times \text{age in y.}) - 2.49$
- $FVC = (0.0576 \times \text{height in m.} \times 100) - (0.026 \times \text{age in y.}) - 4.34$

Chapter 2

Management of respiratory emergencies

29

Managing a resuscitation attempt outside hospital

Resuscitation equipment: See Table 2.1
- Resuscitation equipment is used relatively infrequently. Staff must know where to find equipment and be trained to use the equipment to a level appropriate to the individual's expected role.
- Each practice should have a named individual with responsibility for checking the state of readiness of all resuscitation drugs and equipment, on a regular basis, ideally once a week. In common with drugs, disposable items like the adhesive electrodes have a finite shelf-life and will require replacement from time to time if unused.

Training: Training and practice are necessary to acquire skill in resuscitation techniques. Resuscitation skills decline rapidly and updates and retraining using manikins are necessary every 6–12mo. to maintain adequate skill levels. Level of resuscitation skill needed by different members of the primary health care team differs according to the individual's role:
- All those in direct contact with patients should be trained in basic life support (BLS) and related resuscitation skills e.g. the recovery position
- Doctors, nurses and other paramedical workers (e.g. physiotherapists) should be able to use an automatic external defibrillator (AED). Other personnel (e.g. receptionists) may also be trained to use an AED.

Basic life support: adults 📖 p.34; children 📖 p.40

The recovery position: 📖 p.46

Advanced life support: adults 📖 p.38; children 📖 p.44

Performance management
- Accurate records of all resuscitation attempts and electronic data stored by most AEDs during a resuscitation attempt should be kept for audit, training and medico-legal reasons.
- The responsibility for this rests with the most senior member of the practice team involved.
- Process and outcome of all resuscitation attempts should be audited – at practice and PCO level – to allow deficiencies to be addressed, and examples of good practice to be shared.

Further information
Resuscitation Council (UK) Cardiopulmonary resuscitation guidance for clinical practice and training in primary care (2001)
🖥 www.resus.org.uk

GP Notes: ⚠ Importance of resuscitation training

- Ventricular fibrillation complicating acute MI is the most common cause of cardiac arrest that members of the primary health care team will encounter.
- Success is greatest when the event is witnessed and attempted defibrillation is performed with the minimum of delay.
- It is unacceptable for patients who sustain a cardiopulmonary arrest to await the arrival of the ambulance service before basic resuscitation is performed and a defibrillator is available.

Table 2.1 Resuscitation equipment needed

Equipment	Notes
Defibrillator with electrodes and razor	An automated external defibrillator should be available wherever and whenever sick patients are seen. Regular maintenance is needed even if the machine is not used. After the machine is used the manufacturer's instructions should be followed to return it to a state of readiness with minimum delay.
Pocket mask with 1-way valve	All personnel should be trained to use one.
Oro-pharyngeal airway	Suitable for use by those appropriately trained. Keep a range of sizes available.
Oxygen and mask with reservoir bag	Should be available wherever possible. Oxygen cylinders need regular maintenance – follow national safety standards.
Suction	Simple, mechanical, portable, hand-held suction devices are recommended.
Drugs	Epinephrine/adrenaline – 1mg IV. Atropine – 3mg IV (give once only) – for brady-cardia, asystole and pulseless electrical activity. Amiodarone – 300mg IV – for VF resistant to defibrillation. Naloxone – for suspected cases of respiratory arrest due to opiate overdose. ⚠ There is no evidence for the use of alkalizing agents, buffers or calcium salts before hospitalization. Drugs should be given by the intravenous route, preferably through a catheter placed in a large vein, for example in the antecubital fossa, and flushed in with a bolus of IV fluid. Many drugs may be given via the bronchial route if a tracheal tube is in place; for epinephrine/adrenaline and atropine the dose is double the IV dose.
Other	Saline flush, gloves, syringes and needles, IV cannulae, IV fluids, sharps box, scissors, tape

31

Ethical issues

- It is essential to identify individuals in whom cardiopulmonary arrest is a terminal event and where resuscitation is inappropriate.
- Overall responsibility for a 'Do not attempt to resuscitate (DNAR)' decision rests with the doctor in charge of the patient's care.
- Seek opinions of other members of the medical and nursing team, the patient and any relatives in reaching a DNAR decision.
- Record that the patient should not be resuscitated in the notes, the reasons for that decision and what the relatives have been told.
- Ensure all members of the multidisciplinary team involved with the patient's care are aware of the decision and record it in their notes.
- Review the decision not to attempt resuscitation regularly in the light of the patient's condition.

Further information

BMA, RCN and Resuscitation Council (UK) Decisions relating to cardiopulmonary resuscitation (2001) 🖥 www.resus.org.uk

GMS contract		
Education 1	There is a record of all practice-employed clinical staff having attended training/updating in basic life support skills in the preceding 18mo.	4 points
Education 5	There is a record of all practice-employed staff having attended training/updating in basic life support skills in the preceding 36mo.	3 points
Education 7	Practice has undertaken ≥12 significant event reviews in the past 3y. which could include (if these have occurred) any deaths occurring in the practice premises	Total of 4 points for 12 significant event reviews
Management 7	The practice has systems in place to ensure regular and appropriate inspection, calibration, maintenance and replacement of equipment including: • A defined responsible person • Clear recording • Systematic pre-planned schedules • Reporting of faults	3 points
Medicines 3	There is a system for checking the expiry dates of emergency drugs on at least an annual basis	2 points

Basic adult life support

Basic life support (BLS) is a holding operation – sustaining life until help arrives. BLS should be started as soon as the arrest is detected – outcome is less good the longer the delay.

Basic paediatric life support: 📖 p.40

1. Danger: Ensure safety of rescuer and patient.

2. Response: Check the patient for any response.
- Is he **A**lert? Yes/No
- Does he respond to **V**ocal stimuli? Yes/No
- Does he respond to a **P**ainful stimulus (pinching the lower part of the nasal septum)? Yes/No
- Is the patient **U**nconscious? Yes/No

If he responds by answering or moving: Don't move the patient unless in danger. Get help. Reassess regularly.

If he does not respond: Shout for help; turn the patient on to his back.

3. Airway: Open the airway – place one hand on the patient's forehead and tilt his head back. With fingertips under the point of the patient's chin, lift the chin to open the airway.

⚠ Try to avoid head tilt if trauma to the neck is suspected.

4. Breathing: With airway open, look, listen and feel for breathing for no more than 10sec. – look for chest movement, listen at the victim's mouth for breath sounds, feel for air on your cheek.

If breathing normally: Turn the patient into the recovery position (📖 p.46), get help and check for continued breathing.

If not breathing or only making occasional gasps/weak attempts at breathing: Get help then start chest compressions.

❶ In the first few minutes after cardiac arrest, a victim may be barely breathing, or taking infrequent, noisy, gasps. Don't confuse this with normal breathing. If you have any doubt whether breathing is normal, act as if it is not normal.

5. Circulation: Start chest compressions if not breathing:
- Kneel by the side of the victim and place the heel of 1 hand in the centre of the victim's chest. Place the heel of your other hand on top of the first hand. Interlock the fingers of your hands and ensure that pressure is not applied over the victim's ribs. Don't apply any pressure over the upper abdomen or the bottom end of the bony sternum.
- Position yourself vertically above the victim's chest and, with arms straight, press down on the sternum 4–5cm.
- After each compression, release all the pressure on the chest without losing contact between your hands and the sternum. Compression and release should take an equal amount of time.
- Repeat at a rate of ~100x/min.

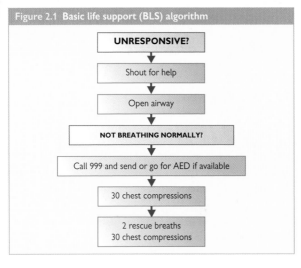

Figure 2.1 Basic life support (BLS) algorithm

UNRESPONSIVE?
↓
Shout for help
↓
Open airway
↓
NOT BREATHING NORMALLY?
↓
Call 999 and send or go for AED if available
↓
30 chest compressions
↓
2 rescue breaths
30 chest compressions

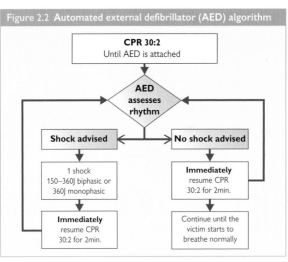

Figure 2.2 Automated external defibrillator (AED) algorithm

CPR 30:2
Until AED is attached
↓
AED assesses rhythm

Shock advised ← → **No shock advised**

1 shock
150–360J biphasic or
360J monophasic

Immediately
resume CPR
30:2 for 2min.

Immediately
resume CPR
30:2 for 2min.

Continue until the
victim starts to
breathe normally

Figures 2.1 and 2.2 are reproduced from the Resuscitation guidelines (2005) with permission
🖳 www.resus.org.uk

Combine chest compression with rescue breaths:
- After 30 compressions open the airway using head tilt and chin lift.
- Pinch the soft part of the victim's nose closed, using the index finger and thumb of your hand on his forehead. Allow the victim's mouth to open, but maintain chin lift.
- Give a rescue breath – take a normal breath and place your lips around the victim's mouth (mouth-to-nose technique is an alternative) making sure that you have a good seal. Blow steadily into his mouth for ~1 sec. whilst watching for the chest to rise.
- Maintaining head tilt and chin lift, take your mouth away from the victim and watch for the chest to fall as air comes out.
- Take another normal breath and blow into the victim's mouth again to give a total of 2 effective rescue breaths. Then return your hands without delay to the correct position on the sternum and give a further 30 chest compressions.
- Continue chest compressions and rescue breaths in a ratio of 30:2.

If rescue breaths don't make the chest rise:
- Check the victim's mouth and remove any visible obstruction.
- Recheck that there is adequate head tilt and chin lift.
- Don't attempt >2 breaths each time before returning to chest compressions.

Chest-compression-only CPR: If you are unable or unwilling to give rescue breaths, give continuous chest compressions only at a rate of 100/min.

⚠ Only stop to recheck the victim if the patient makes a movement or takes a spontaneous breath; otherwise resuscitation should not be interrupted

Use of automated external defibrillators (AEDs) in adults
Program AEDs to deliver a single shock followed by a pause of 2 min. for the immediate resumption of CPR.

If a patient arrests: Start CPR according to the guidelines for basic life support.

As soon as the AED arrives:
- Switch on the AED and attach the electrode pads. If >1 rescuer is present, continue CPR whilst this is done. (Some AEDs automatically switch on when the AED lid is opened).
  - Place one AED pad to the right of the sternum, below the clavicle.
  - Place the other pad in the mid-axillary line with its long axis vertical
- Follow the voice/visual prompts. Ensure nobody touches the victim whilst the AED is analysing the rhythm.

If a shock is indicated: Ensure nobody touches the victim. Push the shock button as directed (fully-automatic AEDs deliver the shock automatically). Immediately resume CPR and continue to follow the prompts.

If no shock is indicated: Immediately resume CPR and continue to follow the prompts.

Use of AEDs in children: 📖 p.42

GMS contract		
Education 1	There is a record of all practice-employed clinical staff having attended training/updating in basic life support skills in the preceding 18mo.	4 points
Education 5	There is a record of all practice employed staff having attended training/ updating in basic life support skills in the preceding 36mo.	3 points

GP Notes:

When to go for assistance: It is vital for rescuers to get assistance as quickly as possible.

When >1 rescuer is available
- One should start resuscitation while another goes for assistance.
- Another should take over CPR every 2min. to prevent fatigue. Ensure minimum of delay during changeover of rescuers.

Duration of resuscitation: Continue resuscitation until:
- Qualified help arrives and takes over.
- The victim starts breathing normally.
- You become exhausted.

Automated external defibrillators (AEDs)
- Modern automated external defibrillators have simplified the process of defibrillation considerably.
- The use of such machines should be within the capabilities of all medical and nursing staff working in the community so ALL practices should have an AED.
- Increasingly trained lay persons are successfully employing AEDs and it is quite appropriate for reception, administrative and secretarial staff to be trained in their use.

Further reading
Resuscitation Council (UK) Resuscitation guidelines (2005)
🖳 www.resus.org.uk

Adult advanced life support

3 basic stages:
- Revive the patient using basic life support (📖 p.34). Basic life support should be started if there is any delay in obtaining a defibrillator, but must not delay shock delivery.
- Restore spontaneous cardiac output, using an automatic external defibrillator (📖 p.35) or manual defibrillator.
- Review possible causes for cardiac arrest and take further action as needed.

Precordial thump: Appropriate if the arrest is witnessed and a defibrillator is not to hand — may dislodge a pulmonary embolus or 'jerk' the heart back into sinus rhythm. Use the ulnar edge of a tightly clenched fist and deliver a sharp impact to the lower ½ of the sternum from a height of ~20cm then immediately retract the fist.

VF/VT arrest
- Attempt defibrillation (1 shock 150–200J biphasic or 360J monophasic)
- Immediately resume chest compressions (30:2) without reassessing rhythm or feeling for the pulse. Continue CPR for 2min. then pause briefly to check the monitor.
- If VT/VF persists give a 2nd shock (150–360J biphasic or 360J monophasic), continue CPR for 2min. then pause briefly to check the monitor.
- If VF/VT persists give adrenaline 1mg IV (or intraosseously if IV access cannot be attained) followed immediately by a 3rd shock (150–360J biphasic or 360J monophasic). Resume CPR immediately and continue for 2min. then pause briefly to check the monitor.
- If VF/VT persists give amiodarone 300mg IV (lidocaine 1mg/kg is an alternative if amiodarone isn't available) followed immediately by a 4th shock (150–360J biphasic or 360J monophasic). Resume CPR immediately and continue for 2 min.
- Give adrenaline 1mg IV immediately before alternate shocks (i.e. approximately every 3–5min).
- Give a further shock after each 2min period of CPR and after confirming that VF/VT persists.

Non-VT/VF arrest
- Start CPR 30:2. Without stopping CPR, check that the leads are attached correctly.
- Give adrenaline 1mg IV as soon as IV access is achieved.
- If asystole or pulseless electrical activity with rate <60 beats/min., give atropine 3mg IV (once only).
- Continue CPR 30:2 until the airway is secured, then continue chest compression without pausing during ventilation.
- Recheck the rhythm after 2min and proceed accordingly.
- Give adrenaline 1mg IV every 3–5min (alternate loops).

Fine VF: Fine VF difficult to distinguish from asystole is very unlikely to be shocked successfully into a perfusing rhythm. Continuing good quality CPR may improve the amplitude and frequency of the VF and improve the chance of successful defibrillation to a perfusing rhythm.

Organised electrical activity: If organized electrical activity is seen during the brief pause in compressions, check for a pulse.
• If a pulse is present, start post-resuscitation care (□ p.46).
• If no pulse, continue CPR and follow the non-shockable algorithm.

Further reading
Resuscitation Council (UK) Resuscitation guidelines (2005)
🖥 www.resus.org.uk

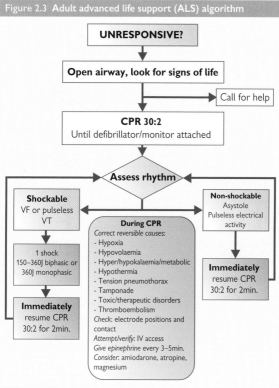

Figure 2.3 Adult advanced life support (ALS) algorithm

UNRESPONSIVE?

↓

Open airway, look for signs of life

→ Call for help

↓

CPR 30:2
Until defibrillator/monitor attached

↓

Assess rhythm

Shockable
VF or pulseless VT

↓

1 shock
150–360J biphasic or 360J monophasic

↓

Immediately
resume CPR
30:2 for 2min.

During CPR
Correct reversible causes:
- Hypoxia
- Hypovolaemia
- Hyper/hypokalaemia/metabolic
- Hypothermia
- Tension pneumothorax
- Tamponade
- Toxic/therapeutic disorders
- Thromboembolism
Check: electrode positions and contact
Attempt/verify: IV access
Give epinephrine every 3–5min.
Consider: amiodarone, atropine, magnesium

Non-shockable
Asystole
Pulseless electrical activity

↓

Immediately
resume CPR
30:2 for 2min.

Pad position: Place 1 pad to the right of the sternum below the clavicle. Place the order pad vertically in the midaxillary line approximately level with the V6 ECG electrode position or female breast (though clear of any breast tissue).

Figure 2.3 is reproduced from Resuscitation guidelines (2005) with permission. Full version available from 🖥 www.resus.org.uk

Basic paediatric life support

Basic life support is a holding operation – sustaining life until help arrives.

Danger: Ensure safety of rescuer and patient

Response: Check the child for any response
- Is he **A**lert?
- Does he respond to **V**ocal stimuli?
- Does he respond to **P**ainful stimuli (pinch lower part of nasal septum)?
- Is he **U**nconscious?

If he responds by answering or moving: Don't move the child unless in danger. Get help. Reassess regularly.

If he does not respond: Shout for help. Assess airway (below).

Airway: Open the airway. Don't move the child from the position in which you found him unless you have to:
- Gently tilt the head back – with your hand on the child's forehead.
- Lift the chin – with your fingertips under the point of the child's chin.

If unsuccessful:
- Try jaw thrust – place the first 2 fingers of each hand behind each side of the child's jaw bone and push the jaw forward.
- Try lifting the chin or jaw thrust after carefully turning the child onto his back.

⚠ Avoid head tilt as much as possible if trauma to the neck is suspected.

Breathing: Look, listen and feel for breathing (maximum 10sec.).

If breathing normally: Turn the child carefully into the recovery position (📖 p.46) if unconscious, and check for continued breathing.

If not breathing or making agonal gasps (infrequent irregular breaths):
- Carefully turn the child onto his back and remove any obvious airway obstruction.
- Give 5 initial rescue breaths – note any gag or cough response.

Technique for rescue breaths:
- Ensure head tilt (neutral position for children<1y.) and chin lift.
- If age ≥1y., pinch the soft part of the child's nose closed with the index finger and thumb of the hand which is on his forehead. Open the child's mouth a little, but maintain the chin upwards.
- Take a breath and place your lips around the child's mouth (mouth and nose if <1y.*), ensuring you have a good seal. Blow steadily into the child's airway over ~1–1.5sec. watching for chest rise.
- Maintaining head tilt and chin lift, take your mouth away and watch for the chest to fall as air comes out.
- Take another breath and repeat this sequence 5 times.

❶ If you have difficulty achieving an effective breath, consider airway obstruction – 📖 p.50

* If the nose and mouth can't both be covered place your lips around the mouth alone as for an older child, or nose alone (close the child's lips to prevent air escape).

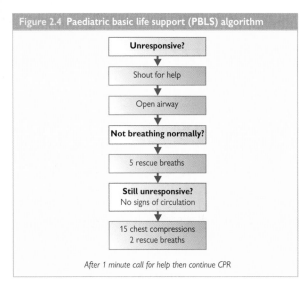

Figure 2.4 Paediatric basic life support (PBLS) algorithm

Unresponsive?

Shout for help

Open airway

Not breathing normally?

5 rescue breaths

Still unresponsive?
No signs of circulation

15 chest compressions
2 rescue breaths

After 1 minute call for help then continue CPR

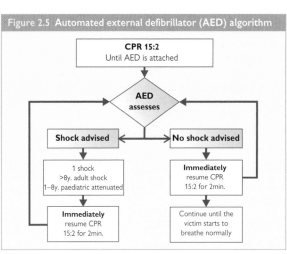

Figure 2.5 Automated external defibrillator (AED) algorithm

CPR 15:2
Until AED is attached

AED assesses

Shock advised

1 shock
>8y. adult shock
1–8y. paediatric attenuated

Immediately
resume CPR
15:2 for 2min.

No shock advised

Immediately
resume CPR
15:2 for 2min.

Continue until the
victim starts to
breathe normally

Figures 2.4 and 2.5 are reproduced from Resuscitation guidelines (2005) with permission. Full version available from ⌨ www.resus.org.uk.

Circulation (signs of life): Check (maximum 10sec.) for:
- Any movement, coughing or normal breathing (not agonal gasps).
- Pulse – child ≥1y. carotid pulse; child <1y. brachial pulse.

If circulation is present Continue rescue breathing until the child starts breathing effectively on his own. Turn the child into the recovery position (📖 p.46) if unconscious, and reassess frequently.

If circulation is absent: or slow pulse (<60 beats/min.) with poor perfusion, or you are not sure:
- Give 15 chest compressions.Then give 2 rescue breaths followed by 15 further chest compressions.
- Continue the cycle of 2 breaths followed by 15 chest compressions.

🔵 Lone rescuers may use a ratio of 30 compressions: 2 rescue breaths.

Technique for chest compressions: Compress the sternum 1 finger's breadth above the xiphisternum by ~$^1/_3$ of the depth of the chest. Release the pressure then repeat at a rate of ~100 compressions/min.
- Children <1y. with a lone rescuer – use the tips of 2 fingers
- Children <1y. with ≥2 rescuers – place both thumbs flat on the lower $^1/_3$ of the sternum with tips pointing towards the child's head and encircle the lower part of the child's ribcage with the tips of the fingers supporting the infant's back. Press down with both thumbs.
- Children >1y. – place the heel of 1 hand over the lower $^1/_3$ of the sternum. Lift the fingers. Position yourself vertically above the chest with arm straight, and push downwards. For larger children use both hands with fingers interlocked to achieve satisfactory compressions.

> ⚠ Stop to recheck for signs of a circulation only if the child moves or takes a spontaneous breath – otherwise continue uninterrupted

Use of automated external defibrillators (AEDs) in children
- Children >8y.: Use the standard adult AED.
- Children aged 1–8y.: Paediatric pads or a paediatric mode should be used if available – if not, use the adult AED as it is.
- Children <1y.: AED use is currently not advised.

If a patient arrests: Start CPR according to the guidelines for PBLS.

As soon as the AED arrives:
- Switch on the AED and attach the electrode pads. If >1 rescuer is present, continue CPR whilst this is done. (Some AEDs automatically switch on when the AED lid is opened).
  - Place one AED pad to the right of the sternum, below the clavicle.
  - Place the other pad in the mid-axillary line with its long axis vertical
- Follow the voice/visual prompts. Ensure nobody touches the victim whilst the AED is analysing the rhythm.

If a shock is indicated: Ensure nobody touches the victim. Push the shock button as directed (fully-automatic AEDs deliver the shock automatically). Immediately resume CPR and continue to follow the prompts.

If no shock is indicated: Immediately resume CPR and continue to follow the prompts.

GMS contract

Education 1	There is a record of all practice-employed clinical staff having attended training/updating in basic life support skills in the preceding 18mo.	4 points
Education 5	There is a record of all practice employed staff having attended training/ updating in basic life support skills in the preceding 36mo.	3 points

GP Notes:

When to go for assistance: It is vital for rescuers to get assistance as quickly as possible when a child collapses.

When >1 rescuer is available: One should start resuscitation while another rescuer goes for assistance.

Lone rescuer: Perform resuscitation for *1 minute* before going for assistance (and consider taking a young child/infant with you to minimize interruption in CPR). The only exception to this is a *witnessed sudden* collapse – as in this case cardiac arrest is likely to be due to arrhythmia and the child may need defibrillation so seek help immediately.

Duration of resuscitation: Continue resuscitation until:
- child shows signs of life (spontaneous respiration, pulse, movement).
- further qualified help arrives.
- you become exhausted.

Cervical spine injury:
- If spinal cord injury is suspected (e.g. if the victim has sustained a fall, been struck on the head or neck, or has been rescued after diving into shallow water) take particular care during handling and resuscitation to maintain alignment of the head, neck and chest in the neutral position.
- A spinal board and/or cervical collar should be used if available.

Further information
Resuscitation Council (UK) Resuscitation guidelines (2005)
🖳 www.resus.org.uk

Advanced paediatric life support

Cardiac arrest in children is rare. Unless there is underlying heart disease, it is usually a consequence of respiratory arrest which results in asystole or pulseless electrical activity and has poor prognosis. Good airway management and providing high flow oxygen for very sick children is therefore important in preventing cardiac arrest.

Basic paediatric life support: Follow the algorithm on 📖 p.41.

Unable to ventilate? Consider foreign body in the airway and initiate airway obstruction sequence – 📖 p.50.

Checking the pulse

- Child – feel for the carotid pulse in the neck.
- Infant – feel for the brachial pulse on the inner aspect of the upper arm.

Once the airway is protected: If the airway is protected by tracheal intubation, continue chest compression without pausing for ventilation. Provide ventilation at a rate of 10/min and compression at 100/min.

When circulation is restored, ventilate the child at a rate of 12–20 breaths/min.

Adrenaline (epinephrine) dose

- Intravenous or interosseous (IO) access – 10mcgm/kg epinephrine (0.1ml/kg of 1:10,000 solution).
- If circulatory access is not present, and can't be quickly obtained, but the child has a tracheal tube in place, consider giving adrenaline 100mcgm/kg via the tracheal tube (1ml/kg of 1:10,000 or 0.1ml/kg of 1:1,000 solution). This is the least satisfactory route of administration.

⚠ Don't give 1:1000 epinephrine IV or IO.

VF/Pulseless VT: Less common in paediatric life support.
- Defibrillation:
  - Give 1 shock of 4J/kg or
  - If using an AED for a child of 1–8y. deliver a paediatric attenuated adult shock energy.
  - If using an AED for a child >8y. use the adult shock energy.
- For VF/pulseless VT persisting after the 3rd shock, try amiodarone 5mg/kg diluted in 5% dextrose.

Bradycardia: When bradycardia is unresponsive to improved ventilation and circulatory support, try atropine 20mcgm/kg (maximum dose 600mcgm; minimum dose 100mcgm).

Magnesium: Magnesium treatment is indicated in children with documented hypomagnesemia or with polymorphic VT ('torsade de pointes'), regardless of cause. Give IV magnesium sulphate over several minutes at a dose of 25–50mg/kg (to a maximum of 2g).

Intravenous fluids: In situations where the cardiac arrest has resulted from circulatory failure, a standard (20ml/kg) bolus of crystalloid fluid should be given if there is no response to the initial dose of epinephrine.

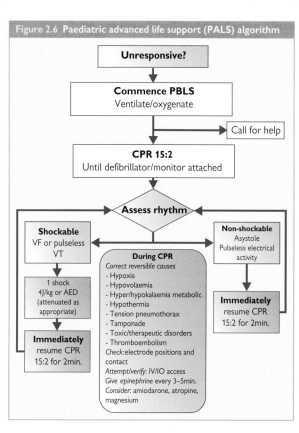

Figure 2.6 Paediatric advanced life support (PALS) algorithm

Unresponsive?

Commence PBLS
Ventilate/oxygenate

Call for help

CPR 15:2
Until defibrillator/monitor attached

Assess rhythm

Shockable
VF or pulseless VT

1 shock
4J/kg or AED
(attenuated as appropriate)

Immediately
resume CPR
15:2 for 2min.

During CPR
Correct reversible causes
- Hypoxia
- Hypovolaemia
- Hyper/hypokalaemia metabolic
- Hypothermia
- Tension pneumothorax
- Tamponade
- Toxic/therapeutic disorders
- Thromboembolism
Check: electrode positions and contact
Attempt/verify: IV/IO access
Give epinephrine every 3–5min.
Consider: amiodarone, atropine, magnesium

Non-shockable
Asystole
Pulseless electrical activity

Immediately
resume CPR
15:2 for 2min.

GP Notes: Estimating the weight of a child for drug/fluid doses

- May not be necessary – use a recent weight from the parent-held child record if available.
- Otherwise for children > 1y., weight (in kg) ≈ 2x (age + 4).

Figure 2.6 is reproduced from the Resuscitation Guidelines (2005) with permission from the Resuscitation council (UK) 🖳 www.resus.org.uk

Recovery position

When circulation and breathing have been restored, it is important to:
- Maintain a good airway.
- Ensure the tongue does not cause obstruction.
- Minimize the risk of inhalation of gastric contents.

For this reason the victim should be placed in the recovery position. This allows the tongue to fall forward, keeping the airway clear.

Putting a patient in the recovery position: See Figure 2.7
- Remove the patient's glasses.
- Kneel beside the patient and make sure that both legs are straight.
- Place the arm nearest to you out at right angles to the body, elbow bent with the hand palm uppermost.
- Bring the far arm across the chest, and hold the back of the hand against the patient's cheek nearest to you.
- With your other hand, grasp the far leg just above the knee and pull it up, keeping the foot on the ground.
- Keeping the patient's hand pressed against his cheek, pull on the leg to roll the patient towards you onto his side.
- Adjust the upper leg so that both the hip and knee are bent at right angles.
- Tilt the head back to make sure the airway remains open.
- Adjust the hand under the cheek, if necessary, to keep the head tilted.
- Check breathing regularly.

⚠ Monitor the peripheral circulation of the lower arm. If the patient has to be kept in the recovery position for > 30min., turn the patient onto the opposite side.

The unconscious child
- The child should be in as near a true lateral position as possible with his mouth dependant to allow free drainage of fluid.
- The position should be stable. In an infant this may require the support of a small pillow or rolled up blanket placed behind the infant's back to maintain the position.

Cervical spine injury
- If spinal cord injury is suspected (for example if the victim has sustained a fall, been struck on the head or neck, or has been rescued after diving into shallow water) take particular care during handling and resuscitation to maintain alignment of the head, neck and chest in the neutral position.
- A spinal board and/or cervical collar should be used if available.

46

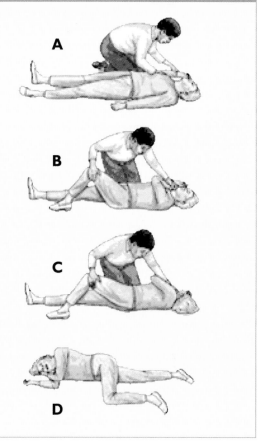

Figure 2.7 Recovery position

The choking adult

> ⚠ If blockage of the airway is only partial, the victim will usually be able to dislodge the foreign body by coughing. If obstruction is complete urgent intervention is required to prevent asphyxia.

Is foreign body airways obstruction (FBAO) likely?

- Sudden onset of respiratory distress whilst eating?
- Is the victim clutching his neck?

Is the victim coughing effectively?

Signs of an effective cough include:

- In response to the question '*Are you choking?*' the victim answers and says 'Yes'.
- Fully responsive – able to speak, cough and breathe.
- ▶▶ *Encourage the victim to cough and monitor*

Signs of an ineffective cough include

- In response to the question '*Are you choking?*' the victim either responds by nodding or is unable to respond.
- Breathing sounds wheezy.
- Unable to breathe.
- Attempts at coughing are silent.
- Unconscious.
- ▶▶ *Call for assistance (e.g. dial 999) and assess conscious level*

If victim IS conscious but has absent/ineffective coughing

- Give up to 5 back blows as needed.
- If back blows don't relieve the obstruction, give up to 5 abdominal thrusts as needed.

Following back blows, or abdominal thrusts: Reassess:
If the object has not been expelled and the victim is still conscious: Continue the sequence of back blows and abdominal thrusts.

If the object is expelled successfully: Assess clinical condition (including abdominal examination if abdominal thrusts used). If there is any suspicion part of the object is still in the respiratory tract or there are any intrabdominal injuries as a result of abdominal thrusts, refer to A&E for assessment.

If the victim becomes UNCONSCIOUS:

- Support the victim carefully to the ground.
- Immediately call an ambulance.
- Begin CPR (📖 p.36) with 30 chest compressions at a rate of 100/min. – even if carotid pulse is present.

Foreign body in the throat: Occurs after eating – fish bone or food bolus are most common. Can cause severe discomfort, distress and inability to swallow saliva.

Management: Refer immediately to A&E or ENT for investigation (lateral neck Xray ± laryngoscopy). Most fish bones have passed and the discomfort comes from mucosal trauma. Food boluses often pass spontaneously (especially if the patient is given a smooth muscle relaxant) but occasionally need removal under GA.

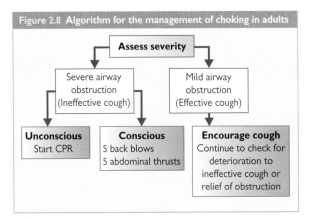

Figure 2.8 Algorithm for the management of choking in adults

Assess severity

Severe airway obstruction (Ineffective cough)

Mild airway obstruction (Effective cough)

Unconscious
Start CPR

Conscious
5 back blows
5 abdominal thrusts

Encourage cough
Continue to check for deterioration to ineffective cough or relief of obstruction

Back blows for adults
- Stand to the side and slightly behind the victim
- Support the chest with 1 hand and lean the victim well forwards so that when the obstructing object is dislodged it comes out of the mouth
- Give up to 5 sharp blows between the shoulder blades with the heel of the other hand.

Abdominal thrusts for adults
- Stand behind the victim and put both arms around the upper part of the abdomen
- Lean the victim forwards
- Clench your fist and place it between the umbilicus and bottom end of the sternum
- Grasp this hand with your other hand and pull sharply inwards and upwards. Repeat up to 5 times as needed.

Further information
Resuscitation Council (UK) ⌨ www.resus.org.uk

Figure 2.8 is reproduced from the Resuscitation Guidelines (2005) with permission from the Resuscitation council (UK) ⌨ www.resus.org.uk

The choking child

⚠ If the child is breathing spontaneously, encourage his own efforts to clear the obstruction. ONLY intervene if ineffective.

Is foreign body airways obstruction (FBAO) likely? Look for:
- Sudden onset of respiratory distress in a previously well child – often witnessed by the child's carer.
- Respiratory distress associated with coughing, gagging or stridor.
- Recent history of playing with or eating small objects.

Is the child coughing effectively?
Signs of an effective cough include
- Fully responsive – crying or verbal response to questions.
- Loud cough and able to take a breath before coughing.
- ▶▶ *Encourage the child to cough and monitor*

Signs of an ineffective cough include
- Unable to vocalize.
- Quiet or silent cough.
- Unable to breathe ± cyanosis.
- Decreasing level of consciousness.
- ▶▶ *Call for assistance (e.g. dial 999) and assess conscious level*

If the child IS conscious but has absent/ineffective coughing
Give up to 5 back blows as needed. If back blows don't relieve the obstruction, give up to 5 chest thrusts (infants <1y.) *or* up to 5 abdominal thrusts (children ≥ 1y.) as needed. Then reassess:
- *If the object has <u>not</u> been expelled and the victim is still conscious:* Continue the sequence of back blows and chest (for infant) or abdominal (for children) thrusts. ❗ Don't leave the child.
- *If the object is expelled successfully:* Assess clinical condition (including abdominal examination if abdominal thrusts used). If there is any suspicion part of the object is still in the respiratory tract or there are any intrabdominal injuries as a result of abdominal thrusts, refer to A&E.

If the child is UNCONSCIOUS: ❗ Don't leave the child
- Place on a firm, flat surface – call out/send for help if not arrived.
- Open the mouth and look for any obvious object. If one is seen, make an attempt to remove it with a single finger sweep.
- Open the airway and attempt 5 rescue breaths. Assess effectiveness of each breath – if a breath doesn't make the chest rise, reposition the head before making the next attempt.
- If there is no response to the rescue breaths, proceed immediately to chest compression – regardless of whether the breaths were successful. Follow the PBLS sequence (📖 p.41) for 1 minute before summoning help if not already there.

If it appears the obstruction has been relieved: Open and check the airway. Deliver rescue breaths if the child is not breathing. If the child regains consciousness and is breathing effectively, place him in a safe side-lying (recovery) position and monitor breathing and conscious level whilst awaiting the arrival of the emergency services.

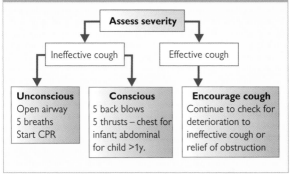

Figure 2.9 Algorithm for management of paediatric foreign body airway obstruction (PFBAO)

Back blows for small children/infants
- Place the child in a head-downwards, prone position (e.g. across your lap). Support the head if needed by holding the jaw.
- Deliver a smart blow with the heel of one hand to the middle of the back between the shoulder blades. Repeat up to 5x as needed.

Back blows for older children
- Support the child in a forward-leaning position.
- Deliver a smart blow with the heel of one hand to the middle of the back between the shoulder blades from behind. Repeat up to 5 times as needed.

Chest thrusts for infants < 1y.
- Turn the child into a supine position with head down (e.g. by holding the child's occiput and laying the child along your arm, supported on your thigh).
- Deliver 5 sharp chest thrusts (like chest compressions but slower rate ~ 20/min) to a point 1 finger's breadth above the xiphisternum.

Abdominal thrusts for children ≥ 1y.
- Stand behind the child (kneel if small child). Place your arms under the child's arms and encircle his torso.
- Clench your fist and place it between the umbilicus and xiphisternum.
- Grasp your clenched hand with your other hand and pull sharply inwards and upwards. Repeat up to 5x as needed.

ⓘ Ensure that pressure is not applied to the xiphoid process or the lower rib cage as this may cause abdominal trauma.

Further information
Resuscitation Council (UK) Resuscitation Guidelines 2005
🖳 www.resus.org.uk

Figure 2.9 is reproduced from the Resuscitation Guidelines (2005) with permission from the Resuscitation council (UK) 🖳 www.resus.org.uk

Anaphylaxis

Severe systemic allergic reaction.

Common causes
- *Foods:* nuts, fish and shellfish, sesame seeds and oil, milk, eggs, pulses (beans, peas)
- *Insect stings:* wasp or bee
- *Drugs:* antibiotics, aspirin and other NSAIDs, opiates
- *Latex*

Essential features: 1 or both of:
- Respiratory difficulty e.g. wheeze, stridor – may be due to laryngeal oedema or asthma
- Hypotension – can present as fainting, collapse, or loss of consciousness.

Other features: All or some of the following:
- Erythema
- Angio-oedema
- Itching of palate
- Itching of external auditory meatus
- Generalized pruritus
- Rhinitis
- Nausea
- Palpitations
- Urticaria
- Conjunctivitis
- Vomiting
- Sense of impending doom

Examination
- *Airway* – mouth/tongue for oedema
- *Breathing* – Chest (wheeze), PEFR
- *Circulation* – pulse, BP
- *Skin* – check for rashes

Algorithms for management of anaphylaxis: Figures 2.10 and 2.11 📖 pp.54–5.

Follow-up
- Warn patients or parents of the possibility of recurrence.
- Advise sufferers to wear a device (e.g. Medic Alert bracelet) that will inform bystanders or medical staff should a future attack occur.
- Refer all patients after their first anaphylactic attack to a specialist allergy clinic.
- Consider supplying sufferers (or parents) with an Epipen or similar which can be used to administer IM epinephrine (adrenaline) immediately should symptoms recur.
- If you supply an Epipen, teach anyone likely to need to use it how to operate the device. Intramuscular epinephrine is very safe.

Further information
Resuscitation Council UK 🖳 www.resus.org.uk

GMS contract		
Medicines 2	The practice possesses the equipment and in-date emergency drugs to treat anaphylaxis	2 points

Action

- If suspected when the initial call for help comes in, call an emergency ambulance immediately – then visit.
- Ask when the initial call is taken if the patient has had a similar event before. If so, ask if he/she has an Epipen or similar. If yes, advise the caller to use it immediately.

On arrival

- Ensure the patient is comfortable – lie down flat ± leg elevation if ↓BP; sit up if breathing difficulty.
- If available, *give oxygen* at high flow rates (10–15l/min).
- *Give IM adrenaline (epinephrine) to all* patients with clinical signs of shock, airway swelling or breathing difficulty. *Dose:*
  - Adult or child >12y.: 0.5ml epinephrine (adrenaline) 1:1000 solution (500mcgm) IM. Give half dose if: pre-pubertal or adult on tricyclic antidepressants, monoamine oxidase inhibitors or β-blockers
  - Child 6–12y.: ½ adult dose – 0.25ml of 1:1000 epinephrine (adrenaline) solution (250mcgm) IM
  - Child 6mo.–6y.: ¼ adult dose – 0.12ml of 1:1000 epinephrine (adrenaline) solution (120mcgm) IM
  - Child <6mo.: 0.05ml 1:1000 epinephrine (adrenaline) solution (50mcgm) IM. Absolute accuracy of dose is not necessary.
- *Repeat* after ≥5min. if improvement is transient, no improvement or deterioration after initial treatment. May need several doses.
- *Give an antihistamine:* Dose of chlorphenamine:
  - Adults and children >12y. – 10–20mg IM
  - Children 6–12y. – 5–10mg IM
  - Children 1–6y. – 2.5–5mg IM.
- *Give hydrocortisone* by IM or slow IV injection. *Dose:*
  - Adults and children >12y. – 100–500mg
  - Children 6–11y. – 100mg
  - Children 1–6y. – 50mg.
- *Give salbutamol* if bronchospasm.
- If severe hypotension does not respond rapidly, start an IV infusion (if available) and *rapidly infuse 1–2l* of saline until BP ↑ (children 20ml/kg rapidly then another similar dose if not responding).
- *Admit the patient to hospital* until ill effects have settled.

🛈 The preferred site for IM injection is the midpoint of the antero-lateral thigh.

53

Advice for patients: Information and support for patients

Allergy UK ☎ 01322 619864 🖥 www.allergyuk.org
Anaphylaxis Campaign ☎ 01252 542029
🖥 www.anaphylaxis.org.uk
Medic-Alert Foundation – supply Medic-Alert bracelets
☎ 0800 581 420 🖥 www.medicalert.co.uk

Figure 2.10 Anaphylactic reactions: treatment algorithm for adults

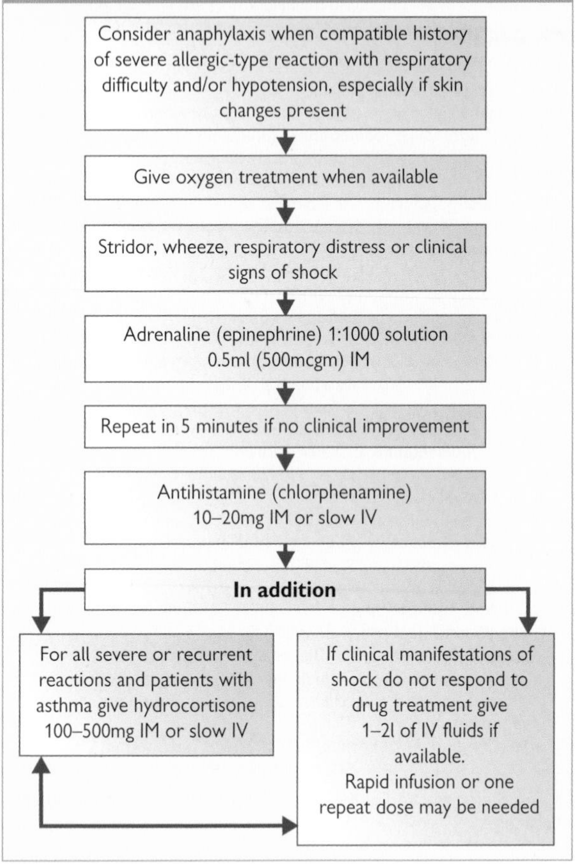

Consider anaphylaxis when compatible history of severe allergic-type reaction with respiratory difficulty and/or hypotension, especially if skin changes present

↓

Give oxygen treatment when available

↓

Stridor, wheeze, respiratory distress or clinical signs of shock

↓

Adrenaline (epinephrine) 1:1000 solution 0.5ml (500mcgm) IM

↓

Repeat in 5 minutes if no clinical improvement

↓

Antihistamine (chlorphenamine) 10–20mg IM or slow IV

↓

In addition

For all severe or recurrent reactions and patients with asthma give hydrocortisone 100–500mg IM or slow IV

If clinical manifestations of shock do not respond to drug treatment give 1–2l of IV fluids if available. Rapid infusion or one repeat dose may be needed

Figure 2.10 is reproduced with permission from the Resuscitation Council (UK).
🖳 www.resus.org.uk

Figure 2.11 Anaphylactic reactions: treatment algorithm for children

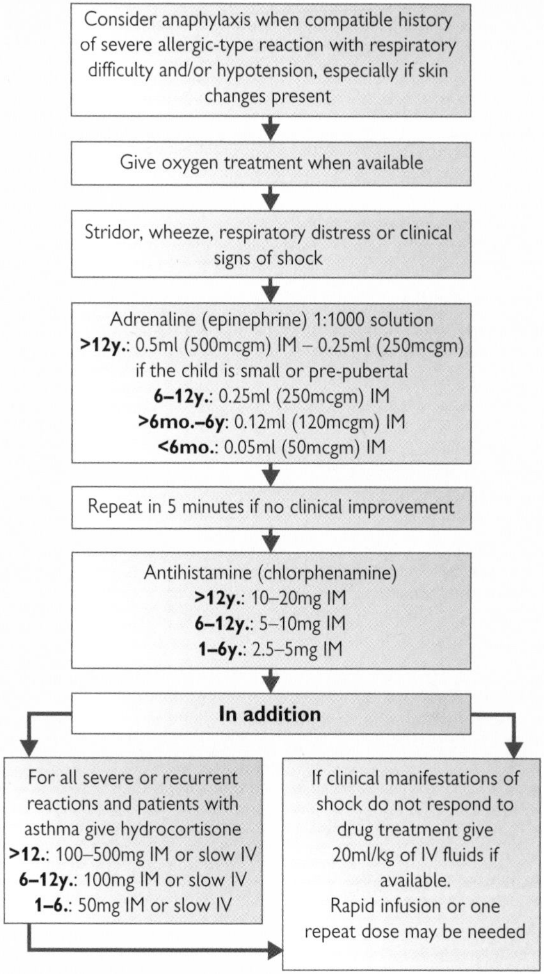

Consider anaphylaxis when compatible history of severe allergic-type reaction with respiratory difficulty and/or hypotension, especially if skin changes present

↓

Give oxygen treatment when available

↓

Stridor, wheeze, respiratory distress or clinical signs of shock

↓

Adrenaline (epinephrine) 1:1000 solution
>12y.: 0.5ml (500mcgm) IM – 0.25ml (250mcgm) if the child is small or pre-pubertal
6–12y.: 0.25ml (250mcgm) IM
>6mo.–6y: 0.12ml (120mcgm) IM
<6mo.: 0.05ml (50mcgm) IM

↓

Repeat in 5 minutes if no clinical improvement

↓

Antihistamine (chlorphenamine)
>12y.: 10–20mg IM
6–12y.: 5–10mg IM
1–6y.: 2.5–5mg IM

↓

In addition

| For all severe or recurrent reactions and patients with asthma give hydrocortisone **>12.**: 100–500mg IM or slow IV **6–12y.**: 100mg IM or slow IV **1–6.**: 50mg IM or slow IV | If clinical manifestations of shock do not respond to drug treatment give 20ml/kg of IV fluids if available. Rapid infusion or one repeat dose may be needed |

Figure 2.11 is reproduced with permission from the Resuscitation Council (UK).
www.resus.org.uk

Acute breathlessness

Attend as soon as possible after receiving the call for help. If there is likely to be any delay, call for emergency ambulance assistance.

On arrival
- Be calm and reassuring.
- Breathlessness is frightening and panic only adds to the sensation of being breathless.
- Direct history and examination to finding the cause as quickly as possible.
- Treat according to the cause.
- If no cause can be found – don't delay – admit to hospital as an acute medical emergency.

Causes: Table 2.2

Acute left ventricular failure (acute LVF): Severe acute breathlessness due to pulmonary oedema. Urgent action is needed to save life.

Presenting features
- Sudden acute breathlessness
- Fatigue
- Cough ± haemoptysis (usually pink and frothy)
- Tends to occur at night
- Some relief gained from sitting/standing

Signs
- Dyspnoea
- Tachycardia – gallop rhythm may be present
- Coarse wet-sounding crackles at both bases
- Ankle/sacral oedema if right heart failure also present
- ± hypotension

Action
- If severe call for ambulance support.
- Sit the patient up.
- Be reassuring – it is very frightening to be very short of breath.
- Give 100% oxygen if available and no history of COPD (24% if history of COPD).
- Give IV furosemide 40–80mg slowly IV (or bumetanide 1–2mg).
- Give IV diamorphine 2.5–5mg IV over 5min.
- Give metoclopramide 10mg IV (can be mixed with diamorphine).
- Give GTN spray 2 puffs sublingually.

Admission: Depends on severity and cause of attack, response to treatment and social support. *Always admit if:*
- Alone at home
- Inadequate social support
- Suspected cause of acute LVF warrants admission (e.g. acute MI)
- Very breathless and no improvement over ½ h. with treatment at home
- Hypotension or arrhythmia.

Table 2.2 Causes of acute breathlessness

Diagnosis	Features
Asthma 📖 pp.60–6	Breathlessness and wheeze. Usually in association with a past history of asthma though can present de novo. Signs of a severe attack include: inability to speak in sentences, tachycardia, pulsus paradoxus, ↑ respiratory rate, use of accessory muscles of respiration, drowsiness or exhaustion.
Anaphylaxis 📖 pp.52–5	1 or both of: • Respiratory difficulty e.g. wheeze, stridor • Hypotension. Other features may include: erythema, angio-oedema, generalized pruritus or itching of the palate and/or external auditory meatus, rhinitis, nausea ± vomiting, palpitations, urticaria, conjunctivitis, sense of impending doom.
Acute left ventricular failure	**Symptoms:** Sudden acute breathlessness; Fatigue; Cough ± haemoptysis; Tends to occur at night; Some relief from sitting/standing **Signs:** Dyspnoea; Tachycardia ± gallop rhythm; Coarse crackles at both bases; Ankle/sacral oedema if right heart failure also present ± hypotension
Arrhythmia	Usually palpitations (though not always) associated with chest pain, collapse or funny turns, sweating, breathlessness and/or hyperventilation. May be a PMH/FH of similar symptoms or thyroid disease.
PE 📖 p.174	Acute dyspnoea, sharp chest pain (worse on inspiration), haemoptysis and/or syncope. Tachycardic and mild pyrexia.
Acute exacerbation of COPD 📖 p.134	Worsening of previously stable COPD. Presents with ≥1 of: ↑ dyspnoea; ↓ exercise tolerance; ↑ fatigue; ↑ fluid retention; ↑ wheeze; Chest tightness; ↑ cough; ↑ sputum purulence; ↑ sputum volume; Upper airways symptoms e.g. cold, sore throat; New onset cyanosis; Acute confusion
Pneumonia 📖 p.152	Breathlessness, cough, fever, sputum, ± sharp, localized chest pain, worse on inspiration.
Pneumothorax 📖 p.172	Sudden onset of pleuritic chest pain or ↑ breathlessness ± pallor and tachycardia.
Choking 📖 pp.48–51	Think of aspirated foreign bodies in any history of sudden onset of stridor or symptoms of respiratory distress.
SVC obstruction	Acute breathlessness, headache worse on stooping, swelling of the face and/or neck with fixed elevation of JVP – admit for assessment.
Air hunger due to shock	Inadequate blood flow to the peripheral circulation – usually associated with ↓ BP (± tachycardia) and peripheral cyanosis.
Hyperventilation	Breathlessness associated with fear, terror and a sense of impending doom.

Hyperventilation

Features: Fear, terror and feeling of impending doom accompanied by some or all of the following:

- Palpitations
- Shortness of breath
- Choking sensation
- Dizziness
- Paraesthesiae
- Chest pain/discomfort
- Sweating
- Carpopedal spasm

Differential diagnosis

- Dysrhythmia
- Asthma
- Anaphylaxis
- Thyrotoxicosis
- Temporal lobe epilepsy
- Hypoglycaemia
- Phaeochromocytoma (very rare)

Action

Talking down: Explain the nature of the symptoms to the patient.

- Racing of the heart is due to adrenaline produced by the panic.
- Paraesthesiae and feelings of dizziness are due to overbreathing due to panic.

Count breaths in and out gently slowing breathing rate.

Rebreathing techniques

- Place a paper bag over the patient's mouth and ask him to breath in and out through the mouth.
- A connected but not switched on O_2 mask or nebulizer mask is an alternative in the surgery.
- This raises the partial pressure of CO_2 in the blood and symptoms due to low CO_2 (e.g. tetany, paraesthesiae, dizziness) resolve. This demonstrates the link between hyperventilation and the symptoms too.

Propranolol: 10–20mg stat may be helpful – DON'T USE for asthmatics or patients with heart failure or on verapamil.

Shock: Due to inadequate blood flow to the peripheral circulation – usually → ↓ BP (± tachycardia), peripheral cyanosis, and ↓ urinary output.

Hypovolaemic shock: Usually due to haemorrhage e.g. GI bleeding, ruptured AAA. *Signs:*

- **Initially:** Tachycardia (pulse >100bpm), pallor, sweating ± restlessness
- **Later:** Decompensation – sudden fall in pulse rate and BP. Young people may decompensate very rapidly. If tachycardic treat as a medical emergency – speed could be lifesaving.

Action

- Lie the patient down flat and raise legs above waist height.
- Call for ambulance assistance.
- Control bleeding by applying pressure if obvious bleeding point (e.g. nose bleed, laceration).
- Gain IV access and (if possible) take blood for FBC and cross-matching – try to insert 2 large-bore cannulae.
- If available, start plasma expander/IV fluids. Give rapidly over 10–15min.
- If available, give 100% oxygen (unless COPD when give 24%).

Cardiogenic shock: Due to heart pump failure e.g. MI, arrhythmia, tamponade. *Signs:*
- Hypotension – systolic BP <80–90mmHg
- Pulse rate may be normal, ↑ or ↓
- Severe breathlessness ± cyanosis.

Action
- Sit the patient up if possible.
- Call for ambulance assistance.
- Treat any underlying cause found e.g. atropine for bradycardia; diamorphine, furosemide and GTN spray (if tolerated) for acute LVF.
- Gain IV access if possible.
- If available, give 100% oxygen (unless COPD when give 24%).

Septic shock: Due to toxins from bacterial infection e.g. meningococcus. *Signs:*
- Hypotension
- Tachycardia
- Peripheral vasodilation or shut down (peripheral pallor and cyanosis, cool extremities)
- Pyrexia
- Tachypnoea
- ± purpuric rash

Action
- Lie the patient down flat and raise legs above waist height.
- Call for ambulance assistance.
- Give IV/IM benzylpenicillin immediately while awaiting transport. *Dose:*
  - Adult and child ≥10y. – 1.2g
  - Child 1–9y. – 600mg
  - Infant <1y. – 300mg.
- If possible, gain IV access whilst awaiting the ambulance and take blood for cultures.
- If available, start plasma expander/IV fluids. Give rapidly over 10–15min.
- If available, give 100% oxygen (unless COPD when give 24%).

Other rarer causes of shock: Admit as medical emergencies:
- **Neurogenic** – due to cerebral trauma or haemorrhage e.g. head injury, subarachnoid haemorrhage
- **Poisoning**
- **Liver failure.**

Acute asthma in adults

Many deaths from asthma are preventable. Delay can be fatal. Factors leading to poor outcome include:
- Doctors failing to assess severity by objective measurement
- Patients or relatives failing to appreciate severity
- Underuse of corticosteroids.

⚠ Regard each emergency asthma consultation as acute severe asthma until proven otherwise.

Risk factors for developing fatal or near fatal asthma
A combination of severe asthma recognized by ≥1 of
- Previous near fatal asthma (see opposite)
- Previous admission for asthma, especially if within 1y.
- Requiring ≥3 classes of asthma medication
- Heavy use of β_2 agonist
- Repeated attendances at A&E for asthma care, especially if within 1y.
- Brittle asthma

and adverse behavioural or psychosocial features recognized by ≥1 of
- Non-compliance with treatment or monitoring
- Failure to attend appointments
- Self-discharge from hospital
- Psychosis, depression, other psychiatric illness or deliberate self-harm
- Current or recent major tranquillizer use
- Denial
- Alcohol or drug misuse
- Obesity
- Learning difficulties
- Employment/income problems
- Social isolation
- Childhood abuse
- Severe marital/legal/domestic stress

Assess and record
- Peak expiratory flow rate (PEFR)
- Symptoms and response to self-treatment
- Heart and respiratory rates
- Oxygen saturation by pulse oximetry (if available)

⚠ Patients with severe or life-threatening attacks may not be distressed and may not have all the characteristic abnormalities of severe asthma. The presence of any should alert the doctor.

Levels of severity of acute asthma exacerbations
Moderate asthma exacerbation:
- Increasing symptoms
- PEFR >50–75% predicted
- No features of acute severe asthma

Acute severe asthma: Any one of:
- PEFR 33–50% best or predicted
- Respiratory rate ≥25 breaths/min
- Heart rate ≥110/min
- Inability to complete sentences in 1 breath.

Life-threatening asthma: Any 1 of the following with severe asthma:
- PEFR <33% best/predicted
- O₂ saturation <92%
- Silent chest
- Cyanosis
- Feeble respiratory effort
- Bradycardia
- Dysrhythmia
- Hypotension
- Exhaustion
- Confusion
- Coma

Near fatal asthma: Respiratory acidosis and/or requiring mechanical ventilation with ↑ inflation pressures.

Brittle asthma
- **Type 1:** Wide PEFR variability (>40% diurnal variation for >50% of the time for a period of >150d.) despite intense therapy.
- **Type 2:** Sudden severe attacks on a background of apparently well-controlled asthma.

Management: Figure 2.12 📖 p.62

Admit to hospital if
- Life-threatening features
- Features of acute severe asthma present after initial treatment
- Previous near fatal asthma

Lower threshold for admission if
- Afternoon or evening attack
- Recent nocturnal symptoms or hospital admission
- Previous severe attacks
- Patient unable to assess own condition
- Concern over social circumstances

If admitting the patient to hospital
- Stay with the patient until the ambulance arrives
- Send written assessment and referral details to the hospital
- Give high-dose β₂ bronchodilator via an oxygen-driven nebulizer in the ambulance

Follow-up after treatment or discharge from hospital
- GP review within 48h.
- Monitor symptoms and PEFR.
- Check inhaler technique.
- Written asthma action plan.
- Modify treatment according to guidelines for chronic persistent asthma.
- Address potentially preventable contributors to admission.

Management of chronic asthma: 📖 pp.110–121

Further information
BTS/SIGN British guideline on the management of asthma (2004) 🖥 www.sign.ac.uk

Figure 2.12 Management of acute severe asthma in adults in general practice

Moderate asthma	Acute severe asthma	Life-threatening asthma
Initial assessment		
PEFR >50% best or predicted	PEFR 33–50% best or predicted	PEFR <33% best or predicted
Further assessment		
Speech normal Respiration <25 breaths/min. Pulse <110 beats/min.	Can't complete sentences Respiration ≥25 breaths/min. Pulse ≥ 110 beats/min.	Oxygen saturation <92% Silent chest, cyanosis or feeble respiratory effort Bradycardia, dysrhythmia or hypotension Exhaustion, confusion or coma
Management		
Treat at home or in the surgery and ASSESS RESPONSE TO TREATMENT	Consider admission	Arrange immediate admission
Treatment		
High dose β₂ bronchodilator: Ideally via oxygen-driven nebulizer (salbutamol 5mg or terbutaline 10mg). Alternatively use air-driven nebulizer or inhaler via spacer (1 puff 10–20x) *If PEFR >50–75% predicted/best:* Give prednisolone 40–50mg Continue or step up usual treatment *If good response to first nebulized treatment (symptoms improved, respiration and pulse settling and PEFR >50%)* continue or step up usual treatment and continue prednisolone	*Oxygen 40–60% if available* *High dose β₂ bronchodilator:* Ideally via oxygen-driven nebulizer (salbutamol 5mg or terbutaline 10mg). Alternatively use air-driven nebulizer or inhaler via spacer (1 puff 10–20x) *Prednisolone 40–50mg or IV hydrocortisone 100mg* *If no response in acute, severe asthma: ADMIT*	*Oxygen 40–60% if available* *Prednisolone 40–50mg or IV hydrocortisone 100mg immediately* *High dose β₂ bronchodilator:* Ideally via oxygen-driven nebulizer (salbutamol 5mg or terbutaline 10mg). Alternatively use air-driven nebulizer or inhaler via spacer (1 puff 10–20x) *ADMIT immediately*

Figure 2.12 is reproduced from the British guideline on the management of asthma (2004) with permission from SIGN/British Thoracic Society.

62

Acute asthma in children

Assess and record
- Pulse rate – increasing heart rate generally reflects ↑ severity
- Respiratory rate and breathlessness
- Use of accessory muscles – best noted by palpation of neck muscles
- Amount of wheezing
- Degree of agitation and conscious level

Levels of severity
Child >5y.: Figure 2.13
Child 2–5y.: Figure 2.14, 📖 p.66
Child <2y.: Assessment of children <2y. can be difficult.
- *Moderate wheezing:*
  - O_2 saturation ≥92%
  - Audible wheezing
  - Using accessory muscles
  - Still feeding
- *Severe wheezing:*
  - O_2 saturation <92%
  - Cyanosis
  - Marked respiratory distress
  - Too breathless to feed
- *Life-threatening:*
  - Apnoea
  - Bradycardia
  - Poor respiratory effort

⚠ If a patient has signs and symptoms across categories, always treat according to the most severe features.

Management
Child >5y.: Figure 2.13
Child 2–5y.: Figure 2.14, 📖 p.66
Child <2y.: Intermittent wheezing attacks are usually in response to viral infection and when response to bronchodilators is inconsistent.
- If mild/moderate wheeze:
  - A trial of bronchodilators can be considered if symptoms are of concern – use a metred dose inhaler and spacer with a face mask
  - If no response consider alternative diagnosis (aspiration pneumonitis, pneumonia, bronchiolitis, tracheomalacia, CF, congenital anomaly) and/or admit.
- *If severe wheezing:* Admit to hospital.
- *If any life-threatening features:* Admit immediately as a blue-light emergency.

Follow-up after treatment or discharge from hospital
- GP review within 1 week.
- Monitor symptoms, PEFR and check inhaler technique.
- Written asthma action plan.
- Modify treatment according to guidelines for chronic persistent asthma.
- Address potentially preventable contributors to admission.

Management of chronic asthma
- *Children <12y.:* 📖 pp.76–83
- *Children >12y. and adults:* 📖 pp.110–21

Figure 2.13 Management of acute asthma in children >5y. in general practice

ASSESS ASTHMA SEVERITY		
Moderate exacerbation	Severe exacerbation	Life-threatening asthma
Oxygen saturation ≥92% PEFR ≥50% best or predicted Able to talk Heart rate ≤120/min. Respiratory rate ≤30/min.	Oxygen saturation <92% PEFR <50% best or predicted Too breathless to talk Heart rate >120/min. Respiratory rate >30/min. Use of accessory neck muscles	Oxygen saturation <92% PEFR <33% best or predicted Silent chest Poor respiratory effort Agitation Altered consciousness Cyanosis
β_2 agonist 2–4 puffs via spacer Consider soluble prednisolone 30–40mg **Increase β_2 agonist dose by 2 puffs every 2min. up to 10 puffs according to response**	Oxygen via face mask β_2 agonist 10 puffs via spacer ± facemask or nebulized salbutamol 2.5–5mg (or terbutaline 5–10mg) Soluble prednisolone 30–40mg **Assess response to treatment 15min. after β_2 agonist**	Oxygen via face mask Nebulize: -salbutamol 5mg or terbutaline 10mg + -ipratropium 0.25mg Soluble prednisolone 30–40mg or IV hydrocortisone 100mg
IF POOR RESPONSE ARRANGE ADMISSION	IF POOR RESPONSE REPEAT β_2 AGONIST AND ARRANGE ADMISSION	REPEAT β_2 AGONIST VIA OXYGEN-DRIVEN NEBULIZER WHILST ARRANGING IMMEDIATE HOSPITAL ADMISSION
GOOD RESPONSE Continue up to 10 puffs or nebulized β2 agonist as needed (max. every 4h.) **If symptoms are not controlled repeat β_2 agonist and refer to hospital** Continue prednisolone for up to 3d. Arrange follow-up clinic visit	POOR RESPONSE Stay with the patient until the ambulance arrives Send written assessment and referral details Repeat β_2 agonist via oxygen-driven nebulizer in the ambulance	

65

⚠ *Lower threshold for admission if*
- Attack in late afternoon or at night
- Recent hospital admission or previous severe attack
- Concern over social circumstances or ability to cope at home

Figure 2.13 is reproduced from the British guideline on the management of asthma (2004) with permission from SIGN/British Thoracic Society.

Figure 2.14 Management of acute asthma in children 2–5y. in general practice

ASSESS ASTHMA SEVERITY		
Moderate exacerbation	Severe exacerbation	Life-threatening asthma
Oxygen saturation ≥92% Able to talk Heart rate ≤130/min. Respiratory rate ≤50/min.	Oxygen saturation <92% Too breathless to talk Heart rate >130/min. Respiratory rate >50/min. Use of accessory neck muscles	Oxygen saturation <92% Silent chest Poor respiratory effort Agitation Altered consciousness Cyanosis
β₂ agonist 2–4 puffs via spacer Consider soluble prednisolone 20mg **Increase β₂ agonist dose by 2 puffs every 2min. up to 10 puffs according to response**	Oxygen via face mask β₂ agonist 10 puffs via spacer ± facemask or nebulized salbutamol 2.5–5mg (or terbutaline 5mg) Soluble prednisolone 20mg **Assess response to treatment 15min. after β₂ agonist**	Oxygen via face mask Nebulize: -salbutamol 2.5mg or terbutaline 5mg + -ipratropium 0.25mg Soluble prednisolone 20mg or IV hydrocortisone 50mg
IF POOR RESPONSE ARRANGE ADMISSION	IF POOR RESPONSE REPEAT β₂ AGONIST AND ARRANGE ADMISSION	REPEAT β₂ AGONIST VIA OXYGEN-DRIVEN NEBULIZER WHILST ARRANGING IMMEDIATE HOSPITAL ADMISSION
GOOD RESPONSE Continue up to 10 puffs or nebulized β2 agonist as needed (max. every 4h.) **If symptoms are not controlled repeat β₂ agonist and refer to hospital** Continue prednisolone for up to 3d. Arrange follow-up clinic visit	POOR RESPONSE Stay with the patient until the ambulance arrives Send written assessment and referral details Repeat β₂ agonist via oxygen-driven nebulizer in the ambulance	

⚠ *Lower threshold for admission if*
- Attack in late afternoon or at night
- Recent hospital admission or previous severe attack
- Concern over social circumstances or ability to cope at home

Further information
BTS/SIGN British guideline on the management of asthma (2004)
🖥 www.sign.ac.uk

Figure 2.14 is reproduced from the British guideline on the management of asthma (2004) with permission from SIGN/British Thoracic Society.

Chapter 3

Diagnosis and management of childhood respiratory problems

Wheezing in the under 2's

Wheezing in children is common and increasing. Up to 20% of children wheeze at some point.

Asthma and viral-associated wheeze: Most wheezing episodes in infancy are precipitated by respiratory infections and will often resolve spontaneously. It can be difficult to differentiate between asthma and non-asthmatic viral-associated wheeze. Asthma is suggested by persisting symptoms and signs between acute attacks and/or a personal or family history of atopic conditions e.g. eczema or hay fever.

Prognostic categories: There are 3 major groups of wheezy children.

- *Persistent wheezers:* ~14% wheezy children. Wheeze as infants and have risk factors for atopic asthma e.g. family history, ↑ IgE levels. Initially have wheeze associated with viral infections. Wheezing persists into school age.
- *Transient wheezers:* ~20% wheezy children. Wheeze associated with viral infection ± ↓ lung function as infants but no risk factors for atopic asthma. Stop wheezing by age 3y.
- *Late-onset wheezers:* ~15% wheezy children. No wheezing before age 3y. Wheezing has started by school age.

Wheeze in the first year of life predicts wheezing later on – 14% of children who suffered 1 attack of wheezing and 23% of children who suffered ≥4 attacks of wheezing under 1y. of age, suffer wheezing attacks aged 10y.

Diagnosis of asthma: 📖 p.70

Management: If the child is compromised by wheezing/shortness of breath, consider a trial of bronchodilators.

- Evidence for effectiveness of salbutamol in the under 2's is mixed.
- There is no evidence that nebulized salbutamol is any more effective than salbutamol delivered via metred dose inhaler and spacer device.
- Oral salbutamol may be useful to avert attacks in children under 14mo.
- Effectiveness of inhaled corticosteroids amongst the under 2's is not clear. Parents report subjective benefits but there is no objective evidence of benefit at standard doses. Higher doses may be more effective.

❶ If there is no response consider alternative diagnosis – aspiration pneumonitis, pneumonia, bronchiolitis, tracheomalacia, CF, congenital anomaly and/or admit.

Bronchopulmonary dysplasia: Extremely premature babies may develop bronchopulmonary dysplasia (chronic lung disease) and be ventilator and oxygen dependent for many months. These babies are often sent home on oxygen via nasal cannulae and may wheeze. They are at higher risk from respiratory infections, particularly RSV. Episodes of bradycardia and apnoea are common. Have a low threshold for readmission.

Further information
BMJ Learning Childhood asthma: diagnosis and treatment
⊞ www.bmjlearning.com
Clinical evidence: Keeley & McKean Asthma and other wheezing disorders in children (2004) Accessed via ⊞ www.nelh.nhs.uk

Diagnosis of asthma in children

Symptoms/signs of a severe asthma attack in children >2y.

- Unable to complete sentences in one breath or too breathless to talk/feed
- Tachycardia:
  - Pulse >120 bpm if >5y.
  - Pulse >130 bpm if 2–5y.
- Tachypnoea:
  - respiratory rate >30 breaths/min. if >5y.
  - respiratory rate >50 breaths/min. if 2–5y.

Life-threatening signs in children age >2y.

- Central cyanosis
- Silent chest (inaudible wheeze)
- Poor respiratory effort
- Confusion
- Exhaustion
- Hypotension
- Coma

Symptoms/signs of a significant asthma attack if <2y.

- Audible wheezing
- Using accessory muscles
- Cyanosis
- Marked respiratory distress
- Too breathless to feed

Management of an acute asthma attack: 📖 pp.64–6

Childhood asthma affects ~5% of children in the UK and the prevalence is increasing. Virus-associated wheeze affects up to 20% of children at some point. Peak age of onset is 5y. Despite increased detection and better treatment of asthma in recent years in the UK, 40 children still die every year from the disease.

Risk factors

- Family history of atopy – particularly mother and/or siblings
- Co-existence of atopic disease – this is also a risk factor for persistence of symptoms
- In pre-pubertal children ♂:♀=3:2. After puberty ♀>♂. Boys are more likely to 'grow out' of their symptoms
- Bronchiolitis in infancy
- Parental smoking – particularly the mother
- Prematurity
- Age at first presentation – the earlier the onset, the better the prognosis. The majority of children presenting aged <2y. are free of symptoms by 6–11y.

Differential diagnosis: Table 3.1

History: History is the cornerstone of diagnosis. Suspect asthma in any child with a history of ≥1 of:

- Persistent or recurrent dry cough – particularly if worse at night
- Wheeze (or noisy breathing)
- Breathlessness
- Tightness of the chest.

Making a diagnosis of asthma in children: Figure 3.1, 📖 p.73

GMS contract

Asthma 1	The practice can produce a register of patients with asthma, excluding patients with asthma who have been prescribed no asthma-related drugs in the last 12mo.	4 points	
Asthma 8	% of patients aged ≥8y. diagnosed as having asthma from 1.4.2006 with measures of variability or reversibility	up to 15 points	40–80%

Table 3.1 Differential diagnosis of wheezing in children

Clinical clue	Possible diagnosis
Perinatal and family history	
Symptoms present from birth or with perinatal lung problems	CF, chronic lung disease, ciliary dyskinesia, developmental anomaly e.g. tracheo-oesophageal fistula
Family history of unusual chest disease	CF, developmental anomaly, neuro-muscular disorder
Severe upper respiratory tract disease	Defect of host defence
Symptoms and signs	
Persistent wet cough	CF, recurrent aspiration, host defence disorder
Excessive vomiting or posseting	Reflux ± aspiration
Dysphagia	Swallowing problems ± aspiration
Abnormal voice or cry	Laryngeal problem
Focal signs in the chest	Developmental disease, postviral syndrome, bronchiectasis, TB
Inspiratory stridor as well as wheeze	Central airways or laryngeal disorder
Failure to thrive	CF, host defence defect, gastro-oesophageal reflux
Investigations	
Focal or persistent radiological changes	Developmental disorder, postinfective disorder, recurrent aspiration, inhaled foreign body, bronchiectasis, TB

71

Advice for patients: Information and support for parents and children

Asthma UK ☎ 08457 01 02 03 🖳 www.asthma.org.uk

Table 3.1 is reproduced from the British guideline on the management of asthma (2004) with permission from SIGN/British Thoracic Society.

Common precipitating/exacerbating factors
- Exercise
- Emotion
- Weather – fog, cold air, thunderstorms
- Air pollutants – smoke, dust
- Household allergens – house dust mite, animal fur, feathers
- Infection – commonly viral URTI, chest infection
- Drugs – NSAIDs, β-blockers

Examination: Is often normal.
- When there are signs, the most common is audible wheeze heard within the chest via a stethoscope.
- There may be signs of other associated atopic conditions e.g. eczema or hayfever or triggering conditions e.g. URTI.
- Rarely, severe asthma may cause impaired growth/failure to thrive or chest deformity e.g. Harrison's sulcus or pigeon chest.

Investigations
In school children: As for adults (📖 p.106), diagnosis can be confirmed using:
- Bronchodilator responsiveness measured with PEFR or spirometry$^£$
- Peak flow variability (and night-time dipping) demonstrated through PEFR diary$^£$ or
- Bronchial hyper-reactivity testing$^£$.

In younger children: It is often not possible to measure airway function in order to confirm the presence of variable airways obstruction. Trial of medication may be the only way to confirm diagnosis.

Expected PEFR in children: 📖 p.25

Viral-induced wheeze: 📖 p.68

Further information
British Thoracic Society/SIGN British guideline on the management of asthma (revised 2004) 🖥 www.sign.ac.uk

---

GP Notes: Measuring peak expiratory flow rate (PEFR) in children

- Use a low-range meter if predicted or best PEFR is <250l/min.
- Ask the patient to stand up (if possible) and hold the peak flow meter horizontally.
- Check the indicator is at zero and the track clear.
- Ask the patient to take a deep breath and blow out forcefully into the peak flow meter, ensuring lips are sealed firmly around the mouthpiece.
- Read the PEFR off the meter. The best of 3 attempts is recorded.
- If the child is having difficulty practise with a whistle or other suitable musical toy.

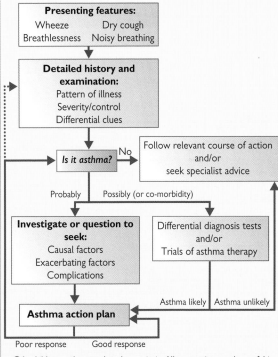

Figure 3.1 Diagnosis of asthma in children

Presenting features:
Wheeze   Dry cough
Breathlessness   Noisy breathing

Detailed history and examination:
Pattern of illness
Severity/control
Differential clues

Is it asthma? — No → Follow relevant course of action and/or seek specialist advice

Probably   Possibly (or co-morbidity)

Investigate or question to seek:
Causal factors
Exacerbating factors
Complications

Differential diagnosis tests and/or Trials of asthma therapy

Asthma likely | Asthma unlikely

Asthma action plan

Poor response   Good response

❶ In children, asthma tends to be extrinsic. Allergy testing may be useful in making a diagnosis of atopy and in seeking causal factors. Absence of allergy should prompt consideration of alternative diagnosis.

73

Figure 3.1 is reproduced from the British guideline on the management of asthma (2004) with permission from SIGN/British Thoracic Society.

Advice for patients: Frequently asked questions about childhood asthma

What is childhood asthma?

Asthma is a long-term condition which affects the lungs. The lungs allow us to breathe, exchanging old air in the body for fresh air outside. In asthma the lining of the lungs becomes over-sensitive. This prevents them doing their job properly. There are 4 main symptoms: cough, wheeze, breathlessness and chest tightness – you may have one or more of these at different times.

Why have I got asthma?

We don't know exactly why you have asthma. We know you are more likely to get asthma if other members of your family have asthma, especially your mother or her relations. Also we know that people with asthma have lungs which react too much to the environment around them. In children more boys than girls have asthma, but boys are more likely to grow out of it as they get older.

Why have I developed asthma now?

Asthma can start at any age, even in adults. In most children asthma starts before the age of 5, but sometimes, if you only have mild asthma, it can take a long time for anyone to make a diagnosis.

What should I do to treat my asthma?

You will normally be started on treatment for your asthma and given instructions on how to use inhalers by your GP. Once your asthma is controlled the asthma nurse from your practice will follow you up at least once a year to check you are not having any problems, do breathing tests, answer your questions about asthma, and check you are using your medicines correctly.

The main inhalers used for treatment of asthma are:
- BLUE INHALER (salbutamol) – this is a reliever inhaler which you need to take when you feel wheezy or short of breath or if your chest is tight. It helps your lungs to expand so that it is easier to breathe
- BROWN INHALER (steroid inhaler) – this is a preventer inhaler which you usually take regularly in the mornings and evenings, and may need to continue taking for months or even years. You will not notice an immediate effect after taking this inhaler. It makes your lungs less sensitive and it less likely that you will get wheezy or short of breath.

There are other inhalers that are sometimes used if your asthma is more difficult to control and your doctor will explain these to you.

ALWAYS take your BLUE INHALER with you wherever you go, and make sure you take any other medicine you have for your asthma with you if you go for a sleepover or overnight school trip.

You may be given a SPACER DEVICE to attach to your inhaler. This makes it easier to take your inhaler, and makes your inhaler work better.

STEROID TABLETS (prednisolone) are sometimes also prescribed. They are usually given for just a short period of time to get your asthma under control. Generally they should be taken every day in the morning.

If your asthma is not as controlled as normal or you have new symptoms then you should make an appointment to see your GP. You should also see your GP before you stop any of your inhalers.

What if I do nothing about my asthma?
It is important to treat asthma and follow your doctor's or nurse's advice about taking the medicines (usually inhalers) you are given. Even people with mild asthma sometimes have severe flare-ups and become ill with their asthma. Every year thousands of people are admitted to hospital as a result of asthma attacks and a few even die.

Even if you never have a flare-up, it is still worth treating your asthma as asthma symptoms can make it difficult to enjoy school and leisure activities. The medicines you are given will prevent this happening.

What can make my asthma worse?
Different things affect different people's asthma in different ways. If you know what makes your asthma worse, it is worth trying to avoid it if possible. Things which can make asthma worse include:
- Having another illness such as a cold
- Air pollution such as cigarette smoke or city fumes
- Things you are allergic to such as pollen or animal fur
- Cold weather
- Stress – for example asthma may be worse during exams
- Some medicines such as ibuprofen.

In some people exercise makes asthma worse. Don't avoid exercise but use your blue inhaler before exercise to prevent symptoms and make sure you warm up before exercise and cool down afterwards. Avoid exercising outside in very cold weather and don't exercise if you have an infection such as a cold.

What will happen in the future?
Roughly:
- ¼ who have asthma as children grow out of it
- ¼ have occasional mild symptoms as adults
- ¼ grow out of their asthma as children but relapse as adults
- ¼ have ongoing symptoms.

It is not possible in advance to predict which group you will be in.

Severe asthma attack
Symptoms: Great difficulty in breathing, feeling panicky, unable to talk in full sentences.

Action
- Try to keep as calm as possible as getting worried will make it more difficult to breathe.
- Take your blue inhaler through a spacer if you have one. Repeat every 2–3 minutes until symptoms improve or help arrives.
- Call for help. If you can breathe with difficulty, but speak in whole sentences, you should call your GP; if you can't speak in sentences, are becoming too tired to continue to breathe properly, are becoming floppy or turning blue then call an ambulance.

Management of chronic asthma in children of less than 12 years

Aims of treatment
- To minimize symptoms and impact on lifestyle (e.g. absence from school; limitations to physical ability)
- To minimize the need for reliever medication
- To prevent severe attacks/exacerbations

Management of acute asthma in children: 📖 pp.64–6

GP services: Ideally routine asthma care should be carried out in a specialized clinic. Doctors and nurses involved in asthma clinics need appropriate training with regular updates. Practices should keep an asthma register of affected patients to ensure adequate follow-up and allow audit[£].

Self-management: All children and parents/carers should receive:
- *Self-management education:* Brief, simple education linked to patient goals is most likely to be successful. Include information about: nature of disease, nature of the treatment and how to use it, self-monitoring/self-assessment, recognition of acute exacerbations, allergen/trigger avoidance, patient's own goals of treatment
- *Written action plan:* Focus on individual needs. Include information about features which indicate when asthma is worsening and what to do under those circumstances. Action plans ↓ morbidity and health costs from asthma[C]
- *PEFR monitoring:* For older children (at least school age), record PEFR at asthma review and if acute exacerbation. Home monitoring in combination with an action plan can be useful, especially for children with severe asthma, brittle asthma (i.e. rapid development of acute asthma attacks) and for those who are poor perceivers of their symptoms. Peak flow diary – 📖 p.105.

Reviews and monitoring[£]: Frequency depends on needs. Aim to review all patients with asthma at least annually and more frequently if stepping up or stepping down treatment.
- Check symptoms since last seen. Use objective measures e.g. RCP 3 questions or Revised Jones Morbidity Index – Box 3.1.
- Record smoking status of parents of children with asthma and older children with asthma – advise smokers to stop[£].
- Record any exacerbations/acute attacks since last seen.
- Check medication – use, concordance (prescription count), inhaler technique, problems, side-effects.
- Influenza vaccination is not included in the QoF for under 16's with asthma, but may become a requirement in future. Consider for all children >6mo. with asthma.
- Review objective measures of lung function e.g. home PEFR chart (📖 p.105), PEFR at review.
- Address any problems or queries and educate about asthma.
- Agree management goals and date for further review.

Advice for Patients: Self-help tips

Smoking: Smoking may ↑ symptoms of asthma – children who smoke and have asthma should stop. Cigarette smoke from parents of children with asthma can also make the children's symptoms worse and all parents of children with asthma should try to stop smoking, or at least refrain from smoking in the home and in the child's presence.

Weight: There is some evidence that weight loss in children who are overweight improves asthma control.

Allergen avoidance
House dust mite: There is little evidence that reducing house dust mite results in improvement of asthma. If you really want to try to exclude house dust mite you need to:
- Regularly vacuum the house to create a dust free zone using a powerful vacuum cleaner with special dust filter
- Fit complete barrier bed coverings, remove carpets, and remove soft toys from the bed
- Wash all bed linen at a high temperature regularly and apply acaricides to soft furnishings
- Dehumidify the home.

There is no evidence that air ionizers have any beneficial effect.

Pets: There is no evidence that removing pets from a home results in improved symptoms but many experts still advise removal of the pet for patients with asthma who also have an allergy to the pet.

Box 3.1 Objective measures of asthma symptoms: morbidity categories correlate with lung function

The Revised Jones Morbidity Index: *During the last 4 weeks:*
- Have you been in a wheezy or asthmatic condition at least once a week?
- Have you had time off work or school because of your asthma?*
- Have you suffered from attacks of wheezing during the night?

* If the patient does not work/go to school count as a NO answer.

RCP 3 questions: *In the last month:*
- Have you had any difficulty sleeping because of your asthma symptoms (including cough)?
- Have you had your usual asthma symptoms during the day (cough, wheeze, chest tightness or breathlessness)?
- Has your asthma interfered with your usual activities e.g. housework, work/school etc.?

NO to all questions = low morbidity
1 x YES answer = medium morbidity
2 or 3 x YES answer = high morbidity

ⓘ These questionnaires are not designed for use during an acute attack.

Drug therapy: Use a stepwise approach (Figures 3.2 and 3.3). Start at the step most appropriate to the initial severity of symptoms. The aim is to achieve early control of the condition and then to ↓ treatment by stepping down.

⚠ **Exacerbations:** Children still die of asthma – step up rapidly during exacerbations, step down slowly. A rescue course of prednisolone 30–40mg od for 1–2wk. may be needed at any step and any time.

Stepping down: Review and consider stepping down at intervals ≥3mo. Maintain on the lowest dose of inhaled steroid controlling symptoms. When reducing steroids, cut dose by 25–50% each time.

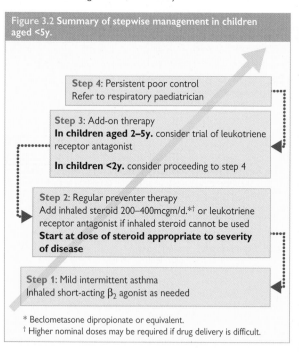

Figure 3.2 **Summary of stepwise management in children aged <5y.**

Step 4: Persistent poor control
Refer to respiratory paediatrician

Step 3: Add-on therrapy
In children aged 2–5y. consider trial of leukotriene receptor antagonist

In children <2y. consider proceeding to step 4

Step 2: Regular preventer therapy
Add inhaled steroid 200–400mcgm/d.*† or leukotriene receptor antagonist if inhaled steroid cannot be used
Start at dose of steroid appropriate to severity of disease

Step 1: Mild intermittent asthma
Inhaled short-acting β_2 agonist as needed

* Beclometasone dipropionate or equivalent.
† Higher nominal doses may be required if drug delivery is difficult.

Figure 3.2 is reproduced from the British guideline on the management of asthma (2004) with permission from SIGN/British Thoracic Society.

Figure 3.3 Summary of stepwise management in children aged 5–12y.

Step 5: Continuous or frequent use of oral steroids
Use daily steroid tablet in lowest dose providing adequate control
Maintain high-dose inhaled steroid at 800mcgm/d.*
Refer patient for respiratory paediatrics opinion

Step 4: Persistent poor control
Increase inhaled steroid to 800mcgm/d.*

Step 3: Add-on therrapy
• Add inhaled long-acting β₂ agonist (LABA)
• Assess control of asthma:
  – Good response to LABA – continue LABA
  – Benefit from LABA but control still inadequate – continue LABA and ↑ inhaled steroid dose to 400mcgm/d.*
  – No response to LABA – stop LABA and ↑ inhaled steroid dose to 400mcgm/d.* If control is still inadequate, institute trial of other therapies e.g. leukotriene receptor antagonists or SR theophylline

Step 2: Regular preventer therapy
Add inhaled steroid 200–400mcgm/d.* (or other preventer drug if inhaled steroid cannot be used)
200mcgm/d. is an appropriate starting point for most children
Start at dose of steroid appropriate to severity of disease

Step 1: Mild intermittent asthma
Inhaled short-acting β₂ agonist as needed

* Beclometasone dipropionate or equivalent.

All doses given refer to beclometasone dipropionate (BDP) administered via metred dose inhaler. For other drugs/formulations adjust dose accordingly (see BNF Section 3).

Figure 3.3 is reproduced from the British guideline on the management of asthma (2004) with permission from SIGN/British Thoracic Society.

Selection of inhaler device
- If possible use a metred dose inhaler (MDI).
- Inadequate technique may be mistaken for drug failure.
- Emphasize patients must inhale slowly and hold their breath for 10sec. after inhalation.
- Demonstrate inhaler technique before prescribing and check at follow-ups.
- Spacers or breath-activated devices are useful for children who find activation difficult and essential for children <10y.
- Dry powder inhalers are an alternative for older children.

Drugs: *BNF 3.1, 3.2 & 3.3.*

Short-acting β₂ agonists: E.g. salbutamol. Use for relieving acute bronchospasm and before exercise for exercise-induced wheeze. Work more quickly and/or with fewer side-effects than alternatives. Use prn unless shown to benefit from regular dosing. Using ≥ canister/mo. or >10–12 puffs/d. is a marker of poorly controlled asthma. Side-effects include tachycardia, hyperactivity and rarely hypokalaemia with large doses.

Inhaled corticosteroids: Most effective preventer for achieving overall treatment goals. Usual dose is 200–400mcgm of beclometasone/d. – this dose has no effect on the child's growth. May be beneficial even for children with mild asthma. Consider if:
- Exacerbations of asthma in the last 2y.
- Using inhaled β₂ agonists > 3x/wk.
- Symptomatic ≥ 3x/wk. or ≥ 1 night/wk.

Oral steroids: Use to treat acute exacerbations. A rescue course of prednisolone 30–40mg od for 1–2wk. may be needed at any step and any time. Don't prescribe long-term oral steroids except under consultant supervision. Prescribing steroids – ☐ p.116.

Add-on therapy: Before initiating a new drug, check compliance, inhaler technique and eliminate trigger factors.
- *Long-acting β₂ agonists:* Inhaled preparations (e.g.salmeterol 50mcgm bd for children >4y.) improve lung function/symptoms. Do not use without inhaled steroids. Only continue if of demonstrable benefit.
- *Theophylline:* ↑lung function/↓symptoms. Side-effects are common.
- *Leukotriene receptor antagonists:* e.g. montelukast. Provide improvement in symptoms and lung function and ↓ exacerbations.

Inhaled nedocromil: is a mast cell stabilizer which ↓ asthma symptoms and severity, bronchodilator use and lung function in children aged 6–12y. when compared to placebo. Dose is 4mg qds, reducing to bd once asthma is well controlled. It is less effective than inhaled steroids and not included in British Thoracic Society stepwise approach at present.

⚠ If poor control check compliance and inhaler technique before altering medication.

Complementary and alternative therapies: Table 3.2

Table 3.2 Evidence for use of complementary therapies in asthma

Evidence	Therapy	
Inconclusive but some evidence of benefit	• Acupuncture[C] • Physical training[C] • Immunotherapy[C] – only in specialized clinics	• Breathing exercises[C] • Herbal medicine[S]
Insufficient evidence	• Massage[C] • Relaxation therapies[S]	• Homeopathy[C]
No benefit	• Chiropractic[C]	• Fish oil supplements[C]

GP Notes: Use of spacers with metred dose inhalers

Advantages of using a spacer

- Allows more time for evaporation of propellant so a larger proportion of active drug is deposited in the lungs.
- There is no need to coordinate actuation with inhalation.
- Less oro-pharyngeal side-effects (e.g. thrush, hoarseness) occur with inhaled steroids if delivered via a spacer.

Choice of spacer: Larger spacers are no longer manufactured. Medium – volume devices (e.g. aerochamber) are effective, acceptable and portable. Always supply infants with a face mask.

Use of spacer devices: Inhale the drug from the spacer immediately after actuation as effect of the drugs is short-lived. Spacers should be washed and air-dried weekly to prevent build-up of electrostatic charge affecting drug delivery, and replaced every 6–12mo.

Advice for patients: Information and support for parents and children

Asthma UK ☎ 08457 01 02 03 🖥 www.asthma.org.uk

Further information

Cochrane: Accessed via 🖥 www.nelh.nhs.uk
- Ram et al. Physical training for asthma (2005)
- McCarney et al. Acupuncture for chronic asthma (2003)
- Dennis & Cates Alexander technique for chronic asthma (2000)
- Abramson et al. Allergen immunotherapy for asthma (2003)
- Holloway & Ram Breathing exercises for asthma (2004)
- Thien et al. Dietary marine fatty acids (fish oil) for asthma (2002)
- McCarney et al. Homeopathy for chronic asthma (2004)
- Hondras et al. Manual therapy for asthma (2005)

Thorax:
- Huntley & Ernst Herbal medicines for asthma: a systematic review (2000) 55(11): 925–9
- Huntley et al. Relaxation therapies for asthma: a systematic review (2002) 57(2): 127–31

Psychosocial factors: Asthma severity is associated with life crises and family conflict. When asthma proves difficult to control on usually effective therapy, find out about any family, psychological or social problems which may be interfering with effective management. Family therapy is an effective adjunct to medication in difficult childhood asthma[C].

Referral: Refer to a general or specialist respiratory paediatrician if:
- Severe exacerbation of asthma E
- Failure to thrive U/S
- Unexpected clinical findings e.g. focal signs in the chest, abnormal voice or cry, dysphagia, inspiratory stridor U/S
- Failure to respond to conventional treatment (particularly inhaled steroid >400mcgm/d.) U/S
- Diagnosis unclear or in doubt U/S/R
- Excessive vomiting or posseting S
- Severe upper respiratory tract infections S
- Symptoms present from birth or perinatal lung problem S/R
- Persistent wet cough S/R
- Frequent use of steroid tablets S/R
- Family history of unusual chest disease R
- Parental anxiety or need for reassurance R.

E=Emergency admission; U=Urgent; S=Soon; R=Routine

🛈 This is only a rough guide, urgency of referral depends on clinical state.

Management of children >12y.: 📖 p.110

Prognosis of childhood asthma: Roughly:
- ¼ become asymptomatic
- ¼ have occasional mild symptoms
- ¼ have a remission for ≥3y. but relapse as adults
- ¼ have persistent symptoms.

Factors associated with persistence
- Family history of atopy
- Co-existing atopic illness
- Female gender
- Presentation age >2y.
- Increased frequency and severity of episodes
- Poor lung function

Further information
British Thoracic Society/SIGN British guideline on the management of asthma (revised 2004) 🖥 www.sign.ac.uk
Cochrane: Accessed via 🖥 www.nelh.nhs.uk
- York & Shuldham Family therapy for chronic asthma in children (2005)
- Bhogal et al. Written action plans for asthma in children (2005)
- Gøtzsche et al. House dust mite control measures for asthma (2004)
- Kilburn et al. Pet allergen control measures for allergic asthma in children and adults (2001)
Clinical evidence: Keeley & McKean Asthma and other wheezing disorders in children (2004). Accessed via 🖥 www.nelh.nhs.uk
BMJ Learning Childhood asthma: diagnosis and treatment 🖥 www.bmjlearning.com

GMS contract			
Asthma 1	The practice can produce a register of patients with asthma, excluding patients with asthma who have been prescribed no asthma-related drugs in the last 12mo.	4 points	
Asthma 6	% of patients with asthma who have had an asthma review in the last 15mo. This should include: • Assessment of symptoms • Measurement of peak flow • Assessment of inhaler technique • Consideration of a personalised asthma plan	up to 20 points	40–70%
Medicines 12	A medication review is recorded in the notes in the preceding 15mo. for all patients being prescribed repeat medicines	8 points	Minimum 80%

Upper respiratory tract infection (URTI)

Viral upper respiratory tract infection (URTI): Children have on average 6–8 viral URTIs each year. Peaks in incidence occur when children start nursery, and start or change schools. Caused by:

- *The common cold:* Acute URTI caused by a rhino (30–50%), picorna, echo or coxsackie virus. At any time only a few viruses are prevalent. Spread by contaminated secretions on fingers and droplet infection
- *Adeno and parainfluenza viruses.*

Presentation: Coryza, runny eyes and malaise. The child may also have mild pyrexia and/or a non-specific maculopapular rash.

Management
- Examine to exclude tonsillitis and otitis media.
- If pyrexia but no other symptoms/signs, check urine to exclude UTI.
- Most viral URTIs settle within a few days with paracetamol and fluids.
- Treat complications e.g. tonsillitis, otitis media, conjunctivitis or exacerbations of asthma as necessary.

Influenza: Sporadic respiratory illness during autumn and winter caused by influenza viruses A, B or C. Spread by droplet infection, person-to-person contact, or contact with contaminated items. Incubation is 1–7d.

Presentation
- In mild cases symptoms are like those of a common cold.
- In more severe cases fever begins suddenly accompanied by prostration and generalized aches and pains.
- Other symptoms follow: headache, sore throat, respiratory tract symptoms (usually cough ± coryza).
- Acute symptoms clear in <5d. – weakness, sweating and fatigue may last longer. 2° chest infection is common.

Management
- *Patients at high risk of severe disease:* i.e. patients with chronic lung disease, cardiovascular disease, chronic renal disease, DM, immunosuppression, asplenism or hyposplenism. Consider treatment/prophylaxis with antivirals – 📖 p.148.
- *Patients at low risk of severe disease:* treat as for viral URTI.

Prevention: Influenza vaccine is prepared each year from viruses of the 3 strains thought most likely to cause 'flu' that winter. It is ~70% effective (range 30–90%). Protection lasts 1y. – 📖 p.148.

Sore throat: 📖 p.144

Croup (laryngotracheobronchitis): Viral infection occurring in epidemics in autumn and spring.
- Starts with mild fever and runny nose.
- In younger children (<4y.), oedema and secretions in the larynx and trachea cause a barking cough and inspiratory stridor.
- The cough typically starts at night and is exacerbated by crying and parental anxiety.
- Some children have recurrent attacks associated with viral URTI.

Management: Steam helps (though beware of scalding children). There is also evidence that nebulized steroids can be helpful but most GPs don't carry them. Admit as a paediatric emergency if there is intercostal recession, cyanosis or parents/carers are unable to cope.

🚺 Suspect asthma if a child has recurrent bouts of croup.

GP Notes:

Advice for carers of children with viral URTI

- Most coughs and colds are caused by viruses.
- An average 5–10y. old has 6–8 coughs or colds/y. and sometimes several coughs or colds one after another.
- Common symptoms are cough and a runny nose. Cough is often worse at night and sometimes children vomit after a bout of coughing.
- Other symptoms include: ↑ temperature, sore throat, earache (and/or ↓ hearing), headache, tiredness and/or poor appetite.
- Symptoms are worst in the first 2–3d. then ease over a few days. Cough can persist for 2–4wk.
- Antibiotics don't kill viruses, so are of no use.
- Treatment aims to ease symptoms. Give plenty to drink. Give paracetamol to ease aches, pains and fever. Ibuprofen is an alternative.
- Sometimes 2° bacterial infections develop e.g. ear infection, pneumonia. Symptoms/signs to watch for include: wheeze, persistent earache or ↑ temperature, fast/difficult breathing, non-blanching rash, stiff neck, drowsiness and/or chest pain.
- Advise parents to call a doctor/NHS Direct if worried.

Advice for carers of children with croup

Croup can be frightening. Young children often become worse late at night. Carers may not know what to do and feel helpless.

Explain the natural history of croup: Symptoms may worsen for 1–3d. and then tend to improve over the next week.

Give advice on self-management
- **Stay calm:** Reassure the child. Showing anxiety can frighten the child, ↑ crying/distress, – which in turn can make breathing more difficult.
- **Sit the child upright.**
- **Keep the child cool:** Remove clothing; give paracetamol ± ibuprofen.
- **Try a steamy environment:** e.g. sit in the bathroom with the door and window closed and the hot tap running (keep child away from the hot water). Alternatively try taking the child outside into the fresh air.

Advise carers to call a doctor/NHS Direct for advice if
- Struggling for breath – difficulty rather than noise is important
- Breathing becomes more rapid
- Very restless
- Drooling or unable to swallow
- Colour changes from pink to being very pale or tinged blue.

🚺 Many children are admitted for observation – often for just 24h.

Lower respiratory tract infection (LRTI)

Bronchiolitis: Occurs in epidemics – usually in the winter months. 70% of infections are due to respiratory syncitial virus (RSV) infection. Usually infects infants of <1y. and presents with coryzal symptoms progressing to irritable cough, rapid breathing ± feeding difficulty.

Examination: Tachypnoea, tachycardia, widespread crepitations over the lung fields ± high pitched wheeze.

Management: Depends on severity of the symptoms.
- *If mild:* Paracetamol as required and fluids. Bronchodilators may give short-term benefit. There is no evidence antibiotics or steroids help.
- *If more severe:* i.e. if the child or parent is distressed, the child is unable to feed, dehydrated and/or there is intercostal recession or cyanosis, admit as a paediatric emergency for oxygen ± tube feeding. Rarely ventilation is required.

Prognosis: A proportion of children who have had bronciolitis as babies will wheeze with URTIs as small children.

Pertussis (whooping cough)^ND: Caused by *Bordetella pertussis* infection. Incubation is 7d.

Presentation
- *Catarrhal stage:* Symptoms and signs of URTI – lasts 1–2wk.
- *Coughing stage:* Increasingly severe and paroxysmal cough with spasms of coughing followed by a 'whoop'; associated with vomiting, cyanosis during coughing spasms and exhaustion – lasts 4–6wk. then cough improves over 2–3wk. Chest is clear between coughing bouts.

Investigation: Microscopy and culture of pernasal swabs (special swab and culture medium available from the laboratory); FBC – lymphocytosis.

Management: Erythromycin in the catarrhal stage. Once coughing stage has started treatment is symptomatic.

Complications: Pneumonia, bronchiectasis, convulsions, subconjunctival haemorrhages and facial petechiae.

Prevention
- *Proven contacts:* Treat with erythromycin.
- *Vaccination:* Routinely given in childhood (Table 3.3). Children with a personal/family history of febrile convulsion, family history of epilepsy and children with well-controlled epilepsy can be vaccinated – give advice on fever prevention. Defer vaccination for children with any undiagnosed or evolving neurological condition or poorly controlled epilepsy until the condition is stable – if in doubt refer to paediatrics.

Acute bronchitis: Occurs when an URTI spreads down the airways. Presents with coughing ± purulent sputum. Chest examination is normal unless asthma is precipitated by the infection.

Management: Advise parents to treat the child with OTC cough linctus, paracetamol and fluids. Wheeze may respond to bronchodilator therapy. Warn parents that cough may persist for several weeks.

GMS contract

Pertussis vaccination can be provided as
- An additional service (📖 p.246) – opting out of giving vaccinations to the under 5's results in a 1% ↓ in global sum; and
- A directed enhanced service (📖 p.246) – 2 payments are available for reaching vaccination targets, one for children aged 2 and another for children aged 5.

Table 3.3 Routine vaccination against pertussis

Vaccine	Age	Comment
Diphtheria/Tetanus/Pertussis/ Haemophilus influenzae type b/ Inactivated polio (DTaP/IPV/Hib)	2, 3 and 4mo.	Primary course 3 doses with a month between each dose
Diphtheria/Tetanus/Acellular pertussis /Inactivated polio (DTaP/IPV)	3y.4mo.–5y. (3y. after completion of the 1° course)	Booster dose 1 injection

GP Notes: Children at high risk of severe bronchiolitis

- Premature babies
- Babies <6wk. old
- Children with underlying lung disease e.g. cystic fibrosis
- Children with congenital heart disease
- Immunosuppressed children

Have a low threshold for admission.

⓵ Palivizumab is a monoclonal antibody indicated for the prevention of RSV infection in infants at high risk of infection. Prescribe *only* under specialist supervision and on the basis of likelihood of hospitalization. Give the first dose before the start of the RSV season and then give monthly throughout the RSV season.

Pneumonia: 📖 p.88
Tuberculosis: 📖 p.158

Childhood pneumonia

Presentation: Diagnosis can be difficult in a child as typical signs may not be evident on first presentation. Do listen to the chest again if the child re-presents even shortly after initial assessment. Typical symptoms/signs include all or some of:

- Fever (bacterial cause is likely if <3y. old and fever >38.5°C)
- Malaise
- Anorexia
- Cough ± purulent sputum
- Tachypnoea and/or other signs of respiratory difficulty e.g. expiratory grunt, chest recession. For older children difficulty breathing is more helpful than clinical signs
- Tachycardia
- Pleuritic chest pain
- Abdominal pain due to pleural inflammation and/or mesenteric adenitis
- Focal chest signs – coarse crackles, reduced breath sounds, bronchial breathing. Generalized wheeze is often due to viral infection.

! Always consider chest infection if the child is ill and there is no other explanation.

Aetiology: Community-acquired pneumonia may be caused by:
- Viral infection: 14–35% – more common in younger children
- Bacterial infection: 10–30% – more common in older children. The organism most commonly isolated is *Streptococcus pneumoniae* followed by *Mycoplasma* then *Chlamydia*.
- Mixed infection: 8–40%
- No pathogen isolated: 20–60%.

Differential diagnosis
- URTI ± transmitted upper airways noise
- Asthma or other wheezing disorder
- Congenital abnormality e.g. tracheo-oesophageal fistula

Investigations: Often unnecessary in general practice. Consider:
- Pulse oximetry (if available) to assess severity
- CXR – only if diagnostic uncertainty/symptoms are not resolving
- Blood – FBC (↑ WCC); ESR (↑); acute and convalescent titres for atypical pneumonia.

Management: Table 3.4
- If symptoms are mild, advise paracetamol and fluids and adopt a watch and see approach, or supply with an interval prescription to use if symptoms are not resolving after 4–5d. or worsening meanwhile.
- Otherwise, treat with a broad-spectrum antibiotic. Commonly used antibiotics are amoxicillin or erythromycin (if penicillin allergic or aged >5y. as atypical pneumonia is more common). Advise parents to bring the child back for GP review if not improving in 48h. or worse in the interim.
- If dehydrated, distressed, not responding to simple antibiotics or any complications – admit for paediatric assessment.

Prevention: Pneumococal vaccination is now part of the routine childhood vaccination programme and is given at 2, 4 and 13 mo.

Table 3.4 Indicators for hospital admission	
Infants (<1y.)	**Older children**
Oxygen saturation <92%	Oxygen saturation <92%
Cyanosis	Cyanosis
Resp rate >70 breaths/min.	Resp rate >50 breaths/min.
Difficulty breathing	Difficulty breathing
Intermittent apnoea	Grunting
Grunting	Signs of dehydration
Not feeding	Family unable to manage
Family unable to manage	Family unable to provide adequate observation/supervision
Family unable to provide adequate observation/supervision	

GP Notes: Recurrent chest infection

Consider further investigation and/or referral to look for an underlying cause if a child has a history of ≥2 probable chest infections. Possible underlying causes include:
- Asthma
- Oro-pharyngeal aspiration e.g. due to reflux
- Cystic fibrosis
- Post-infective bronchiectasis
- TB
- Congenital heart or lung defects
- Immune disorders e.g. HIV, hypogammaglobulinaemia, leukaemia
- Sickle-cell anaemia
- Foreign body in the lung
- Right middle lobe syndrome ● – narrow diameter of right middle bronchus and acute angle → poor drainage and recurrent chest infections. Often associated with asthma/atopy.

Further information

British Thoracic Society Guidelines for the management of community-acquired pneumonia in children (2002) ⬛ www.brit-thoracic.org.uk

89

Cystic fibrosis

Cystic fibrosis (CF) is the most common inherited disorder in the UK (prevalence: 1:2500). Median survival has ↑ dramatically and is now >40y. but, of the 7500 CF patients in the UK, 6000 are <25y. old.

Genetics
- Results from mutation of a single gene on chromosome 7 (cystic fibrosis transmembrane conductance regulator) essential for salt and water movement across cell membranes → thickened secretions. >1200 different mutations have been described.
- Autosomal recessive inheritance – 1:4 chance of having a child with CF if both parents are carriers. ~1:25 adults in the UK carries the CF gene (~2.3 million adults).
- Most common in Caucasians – rare in people of Afro-Caribbean origin.

Screening: Several possibilities:
- *Preconceptual screening:* Buccal smears to karyotype prospective parents
- *Antenatal screening:* Chorionic villous sampling at ~10wk. – for parents with an affected child already or where both parents are +ve on karyotyping
- *Neonatal screening:* A national neonatal screening policy using the blood–spot card to test for immunoreactive trypsin (IRT) is already in operation in Northern Ireland, Wales, Scotland and some parts of England, and will be available throughout the UK by April 2007 – Figure 3.4. IRT is ↑ in infants with CF.

🚯 If IRT is ↑, blood is DNA tested for the 4 most common DNA abnormalities. If 1 abnormality is detected a further screen for another 29 or 31 DNA abnormalities is undertaken. As there are many more mutations described, not all gene mutations will be detected so continue to watch for later presentations.

Presentation: Wide range of clinical presentation and severity:
- Neonatal (meconium ileus) ↑ 10%
- Infancy:
  - GI symptoms alone (failure to thrive; steatorrhoea) – 30%
  - Recurrent respiratory infections – 25%
  - Combination of GI and respiratory symptoms – 15%
- >16y. – variety of presentations (e.g. malabsorption) – 10%
- +ve family history or screening – 10%.

🚯 In future the majority are likely to be detected by screening.

Diagnosis
- Screening – see above.
- If clinical suspicion of CF, refer to paediatrics (or general/respiratory medicine if >16y.). A +ve sweat test (Na^+ >70mmol/l; Cl^- >60mmol/l on 2 occasions) is diagnostic as is ↑ potential difference across the nasal respiratory epithelium.

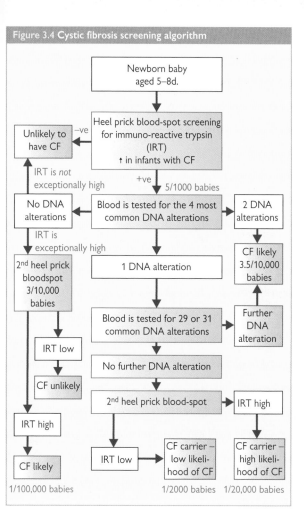

Figure 3.4 Cystic fibrosis screening algorithm

Further information

UK Newborn Screening Programme Centre CF screening
programme and leaflets about CF screening for parents
⌨ www.newbornscreening-bloodspot.org.uk

Advice for patients: Frequently asked questions about cystic fibrosis screening

What is cystic fibrosis (CF)?

Cystic fibrosis is the UK's most common life-threatening, inherited disease. About 1 in every 2500 babies born in the UK has cystic fibrosis. It is caused by a faulty gene which causes organs in the body (especially lungs and pancreas) to become clogged with thick, sticky mucus. Babies with CF may not gain weight well and have frequent chest infections.

Why should I have my baby screened?

The purpose of screening is to identify babies more likely to have cystic fibrosis. You do not have to have your baby screened for cystic fibrosis but screening means that cases of cystic fibrosis are picked up sooner.

What does screening involve?

In the first week of your baby's life, you will be offered a blood-spot screening test for your baby. The midwife will prick your baby's heel using a special device and collect some drops of blood onto a card. The test may be uncomfortable and your baby may cry. Occasionally the midwife or health visitor will contact you to take a second sample of blood from your baby's heel. This may be because there was not enough blood collected the first time or because the result was unclear. Usually the repeat results are normal.

When will I get the result of the screening test?

Most babies will have normal results and you should know the result by the time your baby is 6–8 weeks old.

What if my baby has cystic fibrosis?

If your baby is thought to have cystic fibrosis, you will be given the result by the time your baby is 4 weeks old. Your baby will then be referred to a specialist for further tests to be done to make sure the diagnosis is correct. If cystic fibrosis is confirmed the specialist will start treatment and provide you with more information and support. Babies with cystic fibrosis detected through screening can be treated with physiotherapy, medicines and high-energy diets early on. Although they can still become very ill, it is thought that early treatment helps them live longer, healthier lives.

How accurate is screening?

Screening is not 100% accurate. Some babies will have a positive result and be referred for further testing and found not to have cystic fibrosis. A few babies with cystic fibrosis will not be detected by screening and their cystic fibrosis will be detected later when they get symptoms which need treatment.

Further information for parents

Cystic Fibrosis Trust ▣ www.cftrust.org.uk
UK Newborn Screening Programme Centre Leaflets about CF screening for parents ▣ www.newbornscreening-bloodspot.org.uk

> ## Advice for patients: Frequently asked questions about cystic fibrosis
>
> *What is cystic fibrosis (CF)?*
> Cystic fibrosis is the UK's most common life-threatening, inherited disease. It affects more than 7500 babies, children and young adults in the UK. It is caused by a faulty gene which causes organs in the body (especially lungs and pancreas) to become clogged with thick, sticky mucus.
> - Lung symptoms include troublesome coughs and repeated chest infections.
> - Pancreas symptoms include difficulty digesting food, causing abnormal stools and poor weight gain.
>
> *Why has my child been affected?*
> People with one CF gene, or carriers as they are known, are healthy and show no signs of CF. About 2½ million adults in the UK carry the gene which causes CF – that is about 1 in 20 of the population. For a child to be born with CF, both parents must be carriers. A child with CF has inherited two altered genes – one from each parent.
>
> *What treatment does my child need?*
> You will be referred to a specialist clinic where experts will supervise your child's treatment, monitor progress and provide you and your child with information and support. Your child will need treatment throughout life – usually with physiotherapy, medicines and special high-energy diets.
>
> *What will happen long-term to my child?*
> At present there is no cure for CF but the faulty gene which causes CF has been identified and doctors and scientists are working to find ways to repair or replace it. As recently as the 1930s, children with cystic fibrosis used to die as babies or small children, but now improved treatment means that children with cystic fibrosis are living much longer. It is now normal for children with CF to live to early or middle adulthood and life expectancy is improving all the time.
>
> *If I have one child with CF, what are my chances of having another?*
> - If the parents of a child with CF have another child together, there is a 1 in 4 chance that child will have CF too.
> - If one parent of a child with CF has another child with a different partner, the risk of another child with CF is roughly 1 in 80.
>
> Talk to your GP or health visitor about screening tests available.
>
> ## Support and further information for patients and parents
> Cystic Fibrosis Trust ▢ www.cftrust.org.uk

Common problems associated with CF: Figure 3.5

Management: CF is a multisystem disease requiring a holistic approach to care which aims to maintain patients' independence, improve quality of life *and* extend life expectancy. A multidisciplinary team in a specialist CF centre is best placed to achieve this. Patients usually have direct access.

Treatment of lung disease: Aims to prevent chronic infection as long as possible and later stabilize respiratory infection.

- Exercise: Maintains physical fitness and lung function.
- ↑ *viscosity of secretions:* Treated with physiotherapy ± postural drainage ± dornase alpha (nebulized mucolytic enzyme).
- *Bronchiectasis and infection:* Responsible for most morbidity and >90% mortality. In small children. *S. aureus* and *H. influenzae* are common infecting organisms; in older children/adults *Pseudomonas* infection is common. Treat with antibiotics according to sensitivities. Prevention and control of chronic *Pseudomonas* infection minimizes ↓ in lung function and ↑survival.
- *Airways inflammation and bronchoconstriction:* Managed with inhaled bronchodilators and anti-inflammatories.
- *Pneumothorax* – 📖 p.172
- *Cor pulmonale and/or respiratory failure:* Major cause of death. Cadaveric heart–lung transplantation (50% 5y. survival) or partial lung transplant from a related donor is a last resort.

Maintaining good nutritional state: Patients with pancreatic insufficiency require pre-meal oral pancreatic enzymes (e.g. Creon) and a high calorie diet supplemented with fat-soluble vitamins (A, D and E) – advice from a dietician is essential.

Treatment of complications e.g. DM, osteoporosis

94

GP Notes: Role of the GP

- Communication and ongoing support
- Prescribing routine treatment including O_2 as directed by the CF team
- Providing routine childhood immunizations, pneumococcal vaccination and annual influenza vaccination
- Managing unrelated illness e.g. URTI
- Referral for specialist care e.g. for infertility or genetic counselling
- Certification of illness
- Support of carers
- Terminal care

Advice for patients: Support and information for patients and parents

Cystic Fibrosis Trust 🖥 www.cftrust.org.uk

Further information

CF Trust Standards for the clinical care of children and adults with CF in the UK (2001) 🖥 www.cftrust.org.uk

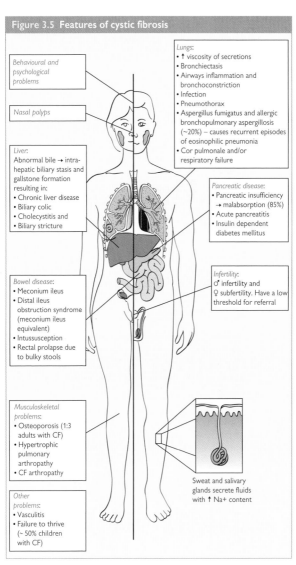

Figure 3.5 Features of cystic fibrosis

Behavioural and psychological problems

Nasal polyps

Liver:
Abnormal bile → intra-hepatic biliary stasis and gallstone formation resulting in:
• Chronic liver disease
• Biliary colic
• Cholecystitis and
• Biliary stricture

Lungs:
• ↑ viscosity of secretions
• Bronchiectasis
• Airways inflammation and bronchoconstriction
• Infection
• Pneumothorax
• Aspergillus fumigatus and allergic bronchopulmonary aspergillosis (~20%) – causes recurrent episodes of eosinophilic pneumonia
• Cor pulmonale and/or respiratory failure

Pancreatic disease:
• Pancreatic insufficiency → malabsorption (85%)
• Acute pancreatitis
• Insulin dependent diabetes mellitus

Bowel disease:
• Meconium ileus
• Distal ileus obstruction syndrome (meconium ileus equivalent)
• Intussusception
• Rectal prolapse due to bulky stools

Infertility:
♂ infertility and ♀ subfertility. Have a low threshold for referral

Musculoskeletal problems:
• Osteoporosis (1:3 adults with CF)
• Hypertrophic pulmonary arthropathy
• CF arthropathy

Other problems:
• Vasculitis
• Failure to thrive (~ 50% children with CF)

Sweat and salivary glands secrete fluids with ↑ Na+ content

Figure 3.5 is reproduced from *The Merck Manual of Medical Information*, 2nd edition, Beers, M.H., Ed. (2003), with permission from Merck and Co. NJ, USA.

Other childhood respiratory conditions

Acute epiglottitis: Bacterial infection causing a swollen epiglottis which can potentially obstruct the airway. Much rarer since introduction of Haemophilus influenza type b (Hib) immunization (Table 3.5).

Presentation: Look for:
- Stridor
- Drooling
- Fever
- Upright leaning forward posture.

> ⚠ If suspected DON'T examine the child's throat as this can precipitate complete obstruction.

Other causes of stridor in children
- Congenital abnormalities of the larynx (below)
- Croup – 📖 p.84
- Inhaled foreign body (below)
- Trauma
- Laryngeal paralysis

Management
- *Child:* Refer urgently but try to maintain a calm atmosphere to avoid distressing the child. Examination should be undertaken in hospital with full resuscitation facilities on hand. Treatment is with IV antibiotics.
- *Adult:* Adult epiglottitis is much less common and less likely to cause complete airway obstruction. Refer for IV antibiotics.

Laryngomalacia (congenital laryngeal stridor): Common amongst small babies. Due to floppy aryatic folds and the small size of the airway in young children. Stridor becomes more noticeable during sleep, excitement, crying and with concurrent URTIs. Normally resolves without treatment but parental concern may necessitate referral.

Inhaled foreign body: Refer to ENT for assessment.

Oesophageal atresia and/or tracheo-oesophageal fistula 1:2500 live births. 5% have oesophageal atresia alone; 5% tracheo-oesophageal fistula (TOF) alone; the remainder have both. Risk factor for sudden infant death syndrome.

Presentation:
- *Antenatal:* At routine USS or following investigation of polyhydramnios.
- *Postnatal:* Cough or breathing difficulties in a newborn infant; choking on the first feed; inability to swallow saliva → bubbling of fluid from the mouth developing soon after birth.
- *Later in childhood:* 'H type' fistulas where there is no atresia but just a fistula may present late with recurrent chest infections.

Management: Diagnosis is confirmed with X-ray. Treatment is surgical. Post-operatively children may have a barking cough ('*TOF cough*') and/or dysphagia – both settle before 2y.

Sleep apnoea in children: Common in children aged 2–7y. in association with tonsil enlargement during URTI. Sleep disruption can cause:

• Daytime sleepiness
• Hyperactivity
• Poor attention span and/or
• Bad behaviour.

If tonsils are big enough to produce sleep apnoea in the absence of infection, refer to ENT for consideration of tonsillectomy.

Table 3.5 **Routine vaccination against Hib**		
Vaccine	**Age**	**Comment**
Diphtheria/Tetanus/Pertussis/ Haemophilus influenza type b/ Inactivated polio (DTaP/IPV/Hib)	2, 3 and 4mo.	Primary course 3 doses with a month between each dose

Chapter 4

Diagnosis and management of adult respiratory problems

Rhinitis

Allergic rhinitis: Common disorder. May be seasonal or perennial. Affects ~15% of the UK population.

Symptoms: Bilateral intermittent nasal blockage; itchy nose, eyes, palate and throat; sneezing; watery nasal discharge.

Signs: Swollen inferior turbinates; ↓ nasal airway; pale or mauve mucosa; nasal discharge; 'allergic crease' on bridge of nose from persistent rubbing (especially in young sufferers). Ask about potential allergens e.g. pollen, feathers, house dust mite, moulds and animals.

Investigation: If symptoms are intrusive and difficult to control refer to an allergy clinic for further investigation.

Skin-prick testing: Identifies IgE sensitivity to common allergens, allowing diagnosis or exclusion of atopy. In most places this is a 2° care procedure though a pilot study has shown it is feasible in general practice. Patients should avoid using antihistamines and steroids before skin-prick testing.

Management

Allergen avoidance:
- *House dust mite:* Evidence that ↓ house dust mite results in clinical improvement is poor[C]. In committed families advise: complete barrier bed coverings; removal of carpets; removal of soft toys from bed; high-temperature washing of bed linen; regular vacuuming and wet dusting; ventilation of the bedroom (open window and door most days); acaricides to soft furnishings; dehumidification.

- *Pets:* Removing pets from a home improves symptoms in some cases. If unable to give up the pet then keep it out of living areas and especially the bedroom; advise regular vacuuming.

Inhalation of steam ± menthol may give some temporary relief from the discomfort of nasal blockage and can be repeated every 2h.

Medication: Table 4.1

Surgical intervention: e.g. referral for nasal cautery or partial excision of the inferior nasal turbinates. Consider if severe blockage and failure of medical treatment.

Desensitization: Desensitization to allergens has a 50–70% success rate. Risk of anaphylaxis is high so, in the UK, provision is limited to specialist centres with full resuscitation facilities. Refer via an allergy clinic.

Further information
British Society for Allergy and Clinical Immunology (BSACI) Rhinitis management guidelines(2000) 🖥 www.bsaci.org

Table 4.1 Drug treatment of allergic rhinitis: *BNF 12.2.1 & 12.2.2*

Category	Example	Notes
Intranasal steroid sprays	Beclometasone 2 puffs bd to each nostril	Effective and can be used safely long term. Takes >1wk. to show benefit – try regular use for >2mo. before abandoning.
Nasal steroid drops	Beclometasone 0.1% 2 drops tds to each nostril	More systemic absorption than intranasal steroid sprays – only use for a limited period e.g. 1mo. and restrict to adults unless prescribed under specialist supervision. *Method of administration:* 'head down' position – kneel with forehead on floor and nostrils pointing skyward. Instill drops and maintain this position for 2min. (📖 p.103)
Topical antihistamines	Azelastine 1 spray bd to each nostril	Can be used as an alternative to topical steroids – faster acting (effect within 15min.).
Topical decongestants	Ephedrine 1–2 drops to each nostril tds/qds prn	Short term (e.g. 5–7d.) for nasal blockage. Of dubious value. Longer-term use may cause a vicious circle – **rhinitis medicamentosa:** vasoconstriction → mucosal damage→ rebound engorgement and oedema →more decongestant use.
Antimuscarinic nasal spray	Ipratropium 2 sprays to each nostril bd/tds	Helps ↓ watery nasal discharge but has little effect on itching, sneezing or nasal obstruction.
Other nasal sprays	Sodium cromoglycate 1 puff to each nostril bd/tds or qds	Less effective than topical steroids but can be useful, particularly in children, to give some relief.
Oral antihistamine	Loratidine 10mg od	Can be helpful used alone or in addition to nasal preparations.
Oral or intramuscular steroids	Prednisolone 10–30mg od or kenalog depot	May be used occasionally for short-term control of severe symptoms e.g. at exam times. A last option.

101

GP Notes:

- Take a careful history of previous treatments tried – OTC and prescribed.
- Often treatments have not been used regularly or for long enough to constitute a fair trial off efficacy.
- Poor technique may also be a factor in failure to respond to sprays and drops – check technique (📖 p.103).

Hayfever: Rhinitis and/or conjunctivitis and/or wheeze due to an allergic reaction to pollen. Occurs at different times in the year depending on which pollen is involved (Table 4.2). The type of pollen that causes hay fever is also connected to where the sufferer lives. In the UK, most hay fever is caused by grass pollen (60%) and silver birch pollen (25%).

Management: Treat with systemic antihistamine e.g. loratidine 10mg od and/or topical steroid nasal spray e.g. beclometasone 2 puffs bd to each nostril and/or eye drops e.g. nedocromil sodium 1 drop to each eye bd. Start treatment 2–3 wk. before the pollen season starts.

When the pollen count is high: Keep windows shut (including car windows – consider pollen filter for the car); wear wrap-around glasses/sunglasses; avoid grassy spaces and mowing lawns.

Vasomotor rhinitis: May be difficult to distinguish from allergic rhinitis as symptoms and signs are similar. Both are common and may coexist in the same patient. Vasomotor rhinitis tends to have less itch and symptoms may be exacerbated by tobacco, change in air temperature and perfumes.

Management
- Try measures for allergic rhinitis as appropriate – often less successful.
- Ipratropium bromide nasal spray helps watery nasal discharge.
- Decongestant tablets e.g. pseudoephedrine used short term may help.

Differential diagnosis: Other causes of similar symptoms include:
- Acute viral URTI
- Acute or chronic sinusitis
- Abuse of nasal decongestants
- Nasal polyps
- Deviated nasal septum
- Foreign body in the nose
- Nasal/sinus tumour
- Cerebrospinal fluid leak
- Vasculitis e.g. Wegener's granulomatosis
- Nasal sarcoid
- Drugs – cocaine, β-blockers, aspirin, ACE inhibitors
- Occupational exposure to nasal irritants e.g. animal workers, farmers, bakers, gloves, solderers
- Ageing/nasal atrophy
- Mucociliary abnormalities e.g. Kartagener's or Young's syndrome
- Immunodeficiency

GP Notes: Frequently asked questions about management of rhinitis

When should I refer?
- Unilateral problems or serosanguinous discharge – to exclude malignancy (refer to ENT)
- Patients not responding to maximal management in general practice (refer to ENT or allergy clinic)
- Children on prolonged courses of intranasal steroids who have slow growth (refer to paediatrics)

Are oral or IM steroids preferable in severe rhinitis?
Oral steroids are preferable as dose is adjustable to severity of symptoms or pollen count, and can be withdrawn in the event of side-effects.

Table 4.2 Predominant pollen types

Jan	Feb	Mar	Apr	May	Jun	Jul	Aug	Sep	Oct	Nov	Dec
Alder Hazel		Elm Willow Ash	Silver birch	Oak	Weed pollen						
				Grass pollen				Fungal spores			

Advice for patients:

Using steroid nose sprays

- Steroid sprays take several days to 3 weeks of regular use to work effectively. Persevere if there is no immediate effect.
- Side-effects of steroid sprays include dryness, crusting and bleeding of the nose. If this occurs stop for a few days and then restart.
- Once symptoms are better reduce the amount of steroid you are using to the lowest dose that controls your symptoms.
- If you use the spray for hay fever, try to start it a week before symptoms usually start, or as soon as you notice the first symptoms.

How to use a steroid nose spray
- Blow your nose and shake the bottle.
- Tilt your head forward.
- Insert the tip of the spray bottle just inside your nostril with the spray-bottle upright. Close the other nostril.
- Sniff in gently as you spray.

Application of steroid nose drops

- Kneel or stand and bend down and forward.
- Stay with the head down for 3–4 minutes after putting in the drops to allow the drops to reach the back of the nose.
- Alternatively, lie with your head tipped right back off the edge of the bed to insert the drops.
- Do not put in nose drops by just tilting your head back as the drops will not coat the upper surface inside your nose.

Information for patients
BBC pollen index ☐ www.bbc.co.uk/weather/pollen
Allergy UK ☎ 01322 619898 ☐ www.allergyuk.org
Patient UK Information leaflets on rhinitis and nose sprays
☐ www.patient.co.uk

Further information
British Society for Allergy and Clinical Immunology (BSACI) Rhinitis management guidelines (2000) ☐ www.bsaci.org

Cartoons are reproduced in modified format with permission from the Patient UK website ☐ www.patient.co.uk

103

Asthma in adults and children of 12 years and above

> ## Symptoms/signs of a severe asthma attack
> - Unable to talk in sentences without stopping for breath
> - Intercostal recession
> - PEFR <50% best
> - Tachypnoea (respiratory rate >25 breaths/min.)
> - Tachycardia (heart rate >110bpm)
>
> ## Life-threatening signs
> - Central cyanosis
> - Silent chest (inaudible wheeze)
> - Confusion or exhaustion
> - PEFR <33% predicted or best
> - Hypotension
> - Bradycardia
>
> **Management of an acute asthma attack:** 📖 p.62

Asthma is a condition of paroxysmal, reversible airways obstruction and has 3 characteristic features:
- Airflow limitation which is usually reversible spontaneously or with treatment
- Airway hyper-responsiveness to a wide range of stimuli
- Inflammation of the bronchi.

Personal or family history of asthma or other atopic conditions e.g. eczema or hayfever makes diagnosis of asthma more likely.

Classification
- *Intrinsic:* No specific triggers – typically starts in middle age.
- *Extrinsic:* Identifiable triggers – typically affects children and young people.

Prevalence: Estimates of prevalence vary widely dependent on criteria used. European Respiratory Health Survey figures:
- 25% adults aged 20–44y. suffer from wheeze
- 15% suffer from wheeze with breathlessness
- 7% have doctor-diagnosed asthma.

There is marked geographical variation. Occupational asthma accounts for 1–2% of adult asthma (📖 p.182).

Asthma in special groups
- *Children <12y.:* 📖 p.70
- *Occupational asthma:* 📖 p.182
- *Pregnancy:* 📖 p.120

> ### Advice for patients: Information and support for patients
> **Asthma UK** ☎ 08457 01 02 03 🖥 www.asthma.org.uk

Further information
British Thoracic Society/SIGN British guideline on the management of asthma (revised 2004) 🖥 www.sign.ac.uk

Figure 4.1 Peak flow diary

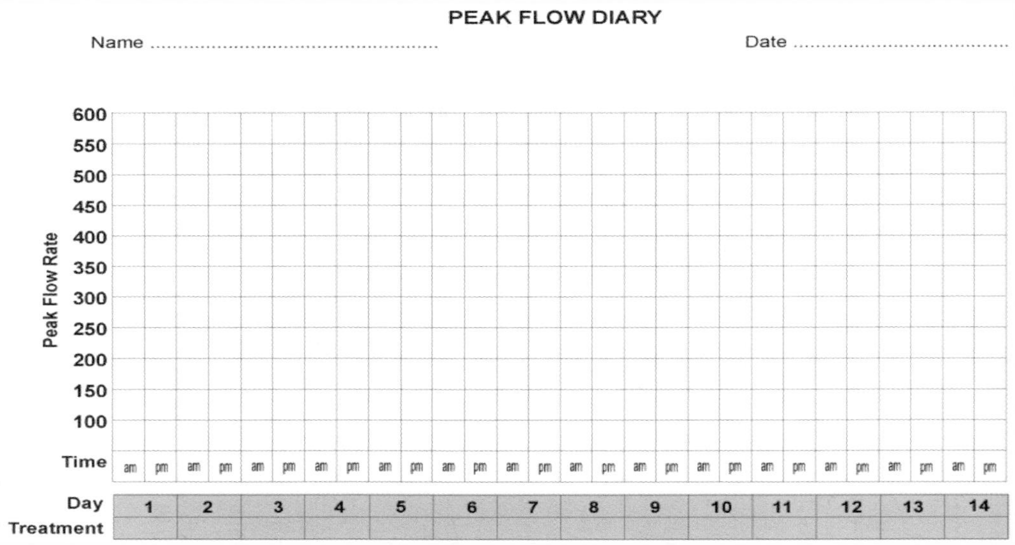
PEAK FLOW DIARY
Name ....
Date ....
Peak Flow Rate
600
550
500
450
400
350
300
250
200
150
100
Time
am pm am pm am pm am pm am pm am pm am pm am pm am pm am pm am pm am pm am pm am pm
Day
1 2 3 4 5 6 7 8 9 10 11 12 13 14
Treatment

Diagnosis of asthma in adults and older children

Diagnosis of asthma can be difficult as people who have asthma suffer from a variety of symptoms – none of which are specific for asthma.

Symptoms
- wheeze
- shortness of breath
- chest tightness
- cough

Typically symptoms are
- variable
- intermittent
- worse at night and in the early morning (when PEFR dips) and/or
- provoked by triggers e.g. exercise, pollen (Box 4.1)

Signs
- **None:** Common if patient is well.
- **Wheeze:** Bilateral, diffuse, polyphonic, expiratory > inspiratory – document in the patient record if wheeze is heard.
- **'Barrel chest':** Signs of hyperinflation ± wheeze in a patient with chronic asthma.

Tests: Use objective tests to confirm diagnosis of asthma before long-term treatment is started[£]. In general practice this involves serial PEFR measurement ± spirometry (📖 pp.24–7).

PEFR
- Normal PEFR + current symptoms suggests diagnosis is NOT asthma.
- Variability of PEFR over time (either spontaneously or in response to medication) is a characteristic feature of asthma (Table 4.3).

Spirometry: Use to exclude other forms of lung disease e.g. COPD. Can also be used instead of PEFR to demonstrate variability (≥15% variation in FEV_1 with a minimum change in FEV_1 ≥200l/min. suggests asthma).

CXR: Consider for any patient with atypical/additional symptoms.

Cough variant asthma: Asthma in which cough without wheeze is the predominant feature.

Differential diagnosis
Localized obstruction of the airways
- Cancer (lung, trachea, larynx)
- Foreign body
- Post tracheostomy stenosis

Generalized obstruction of the airways
- COPD (predominantly irreversible)
- Cardiac disease
- PE
- Interstitial lung disease
- Aspiration
- Bronchiectasis
- CF

GMS contract

Asthma 1	The practice can produce a register of patients with asthma, excluding patients with asthma who have been prescribed no asthma-related drugs in the last 12mo.	4 points	
Asthma 8	% of patients aged ≥8y. diagnosed as having asthma from 1.4.2006 with measures of variability or reversibility	up to 15 points	40–80%

⚠ Patients should not be on the asthma AND COPD register.

Box 4.1 Common precipitating/exacerbating factors for asthma

- Exercise
- Emotion
- Weather (fog, cold air, thunderstorms)
- Air pollutants (smoke and dust)
- Household allergens (e.g. house dust mite, animal fur, feathers)
- Smoking
- Occupational exposure to animal products, wood dusts, grain dusts, chemicals (e.g. isocyanates)
- Infection (commonly viral URTI and chest infections)
- Drugs (NSAIDs, β-blockers)
- Gastro-oesophageal reflux

Table 4.3 Objective tests to confirm asthma

Test	Positive outcome*
Serial PEFR measurements	Demonstrate variability on ≥3d./wk. A peak flow diary is useful – 📖 p.105
Trial of β-agonists	Inhaled salbutamol (2.5mg via nebulizer or 400mcgm via MDI with spacer)→ ↑ PEFR
Trial of steroids	Prednisolone 30mg od for 14d. → ↑ PEFR
Exercise test	6min. exercise e.g. running → ↓ PEFR

*>20% variability from the best or baseline reading, with a minimum change in PEFR of ≥60l/min. is highly suggestive of a diagnosis of asthma.

GP Notes: Measuring peak expiratory flow rate (PEFR)

- Use a low-range meter if predicted or best PEFR is <250l/min.
- Ask the patient to stand up (if possible) and hold the peak flow meter horizontally.
- Check the indicator is at zero and the track clear.
- Ask the patient to take a deep breath and blow out forcefully into the peak flow meter, ensuring lips are sealed firmly around the mouthpiece.
- Read the PEFR off the meter. The best of 3 attempts is recorded.

Expected PEFR: 📖 p.25

Advice for patients: Frequently asked questions about asthma

What is asthma?

Asthma is a long-term condition which affects the lungs. In asthma the lining of the lungs becomes over-sensitive, often to normal every-day substances, resulting in 4 main symptoms: cough, wheeze, breathlessness and chest tightness. You may have one or more of these at different times.

Why have I got asthma?

10–15% of people in the UK have asthma. The number of people is going up but it is not clear why. People probably develop asthma due to a combination of factors. We know you get asthma if other members of your family have asthma. We also know that people with asthma have lungs which react too much to the environment around them.

Why have I developed asthma now?

Asthma can start at any age, even in adults. In most children asthma starts before the age of 5, but sometimes, if you only have mild asthma, it can take a long time for anyone to make a diagnosis.

What should I do to treat my asthma?

You will normally be started on treatment for your asthma and given instructions on how to use inhalers by your GP. Once your asthma is controlled the asthma nurse from your practice will follow you up at least once a year to check you are not having any problems and do breathing tests, answer your questions about asthma, and check you are using your medicines correctly.

The main inhalers used for treatment of asthma are:

- BLUE INHALER (salbutamol) – this is a reliever inhaler which you need to take when you feel wheezy or short of breath or if your chest is tight. It helps your lungs to expand so that it is easier to breathe
- BROWN INHALER (steroid inhaler) – this is a preventer inhaler which you usually take regularly in the mornings and evenings, and may need to continue taking for months or even years. You will not notice an immediate effect after taking this inhaler. It makes your lungs less sensitive and it less likely that you will get wheezy or short of breath.

There are other inhalers that are sometimes used if your asthma is more difficult to control and your doctor or nurse will explain these to you.

ALWAYS take your BLUE INHALER with you wherever you go, and make sure you take any other medicine you have for your asthma with you if you go away overnight.

You may be given a SPACER DEVICE to attach to your inhaler. This makes it easier to take your inhaler, and makes your inhaler work better.

STEROID TABLETS (prednisolone) are sometimes also prescribed. They are usually given for just a short period of time to get your asthma under control. Generally they should be taken every day in the morning.

If your asthma is not as controlled as normal or you have new symptoms then you should make an appointment to see your GP. You should also see your GP before you stop any of your inhalers.

Should I have the flu vaccination?

People with asthma can get flu badly and are more prone to chest infections as a result. A flu vaccination every year will protect you against the strains of flu most likely to make you ill that year. A one-off pneumococcal vaccination will protect you against certain types of pneumonia. If you need more information, see your GP or asthma nurse.

What if I do nothing about my asthma?

It is important to treat asthma and follow your doctor's or nurse's advice about taking the medicines (usually inhalers) you are given. Even people with mild asthma sometimes have severe flare-ups and become ill with their asthma. Every year thousands of people are admitted to hospital as a result of asthma attacks and a few even die.

Even if you never have a flare-up, it is still worth treating your asthma as asthma symptoms can make it difficult to enjoy life. The medicines you are given will prevent this happening.

What can make my asthma worse?

Different things affect different people's asthma in different ways. If you know what makes your asthma worse, it is worth trying to avoid it if possible. Things which can make asthma worse include:
- Having another illness such as a cold
- Air pollution such as cigarette smoke or city fumes
- Things you are allergic to such as pollen, dust or animal fur
- Cold weather
- Stress
- Some medicines such as ibuprofen.

In some people exercise makes asthma worse. Don't avoid exercise but use your blue inhaler before exercise to prevent symptoms and make sure you warm up before exercise and cool down afterwards. Avoid exercising outside in very cold weather and don't exercise if you have an infection such as a cold.

Severe asthma attack

Symptoms: Great difficulty in breathing, feeling panicky, unable to talk in full sentences.

Action
- Try to keep as calm as possible as getting worried will make it more difficult to breath.
- Take your blue inhaler through a spacer if you have one. Repeat every 2–3 minutes until symptoms improve or help arrives.
- Call for help. If you can breathe with difficulty, but speak in whole sentences, you should call your GP; if you can't speak in sentences, are becoming too tired to continue to breathe properly, are boecoming floppy or turning blue then call an ambulance.

Management of chronic asthma in adults and older children

Aims of treatment
- To minimize symptoms and impact on lifestyle (e.g. absence from work; limitations to physical ability)
- To minimize the need for reliever medication
- To prevent severe attacks/exacerbations

Management of acute asthma: 📖 p.62

GP services: Ideally routine asthma care should be carried out in a specialized clinic. Doctors and nurses involved in asthma clinics need appropriate training with regular updates. Practices should keep an asthma register of affected patients to ensure adequate follow-up and allow audit[£].

Self-management: All patients should receive:
- *Self-management education:* Brief, simple education linked to patient goals is most likely to be successful. Include information about: nature of disease, nature of the treatment and how to use it, self-monitoring/self-assessment, recognition of acute exacerbations, allergen/trigger avoidance, patient's own goals of treatment.
- *Written action plan:* Focus on individual needs. Include information about features which indicate when asthma is worsening and what to do under those circumstances. Action plans ↓ morbidity and health costs from asthma[C].
- *PEFR monitoring:* Record PEFR at asthma review and if acute exacerbation. Home monitoring in combination with an action plan can be useful, especially for patients with severe asthma, brittle asthma (i.e. rapid development of acute asthma attacks) and for those who are poor perceivers of their symptoms. Peak flow diary – Figure 4.1, 📖 p.105.

Reviews and monitoring[£]: Frequency depends on needs. Aim to review all patients with asthma at least annually (Figure 4.2, 📖 p.112) and more frequently if stepping up or stepping down treatment.
- Check symptoms since last seen. Use objective measures e.g. RCP 3 questions or Revised Jones Morbidity Index – Box 4.2.
- Record smoking status of patients with asthma and other household members – advise smokers to stop[£].
- Record any exacerbations/acute attacks since last seen.
- Check medication – use, concordance (prescription count), inhaler technique, problems, side-effects.
- Influenza ± pneumococcal vaccination should be offered to all patients with asthma.
- Review objective measures of lung function e.g. home PEFR chart, PEFR at review.
- Address any problems or queries and educate about asthma.
- Agree management goals and date for further review.

Advice for patients: Self-help tips

Smoking: Smoking increases symptoms of asthma. If you smoke you should try to stop. Cigarette smoke from other people in your home can also make symptoms worse so encourage them to stop too – or at least refrain from smoking in the home.

Weight: There is some evidence that weight loss in overweight people improves asthma control.

Allergen avoidance:

House dust mite: There is little evidence that reducing house dust mite results in improvement of asthma[C]. If you really want to try to exclude house dust mite you need to:
• Regularly vacuum the house to create a dust free zone using a powerful vacuum cleaner with special dust filter
• Fit complete barrier bed coverings, remove carpets, and remove soft toys from the bed
• Wash all bed linen at a high temperature regularly and apply acaricides to soft furnishings
• Dehumidify the home

There is no evidence that air ionizers have any beneficial effect.

Pets: There is no evidence that removing pets from a home results in improved symptoms[C] but many experts still advise removal of the pet for patients with asthma who also have an allergy to the pet.

Box 4.2 **Objective measures of asthma symptoms: morbidity categories correlate with lung function**

111

The Revised Jones Morbidity Index: *During the last 4 weeks:*
• Have you been in a wheezy or asthmatic condition at least once a week?
• Have you had time off work or school because of your asthma?*
• Have you suffered from attacks of wheezing during the night?

* If the patient does not work/go to school, count as a NO answer.

RCP 3 questions: In the last month:
• Have you had any difficulty sleeping because of your asthma symptoms (including cough)?
• Have you had your usual asthma symptoms during the day (cough, wheeze, chest tightness or breathlessness)?
• Has your asthma interfered with your usual activities e.g. housework, work/school etc.?

NO to all questions = low morbidity
1 x YES answer = medium morbidity
2 or 3 x YES answer = high morbidity

❶ These questionnaires are not designed for use during an acute attack.

The Revised Jones Morbidity Index is reproduced with permission from Dr Kevin Jones. The RCP3 questions are reproduced with permission from RCP.

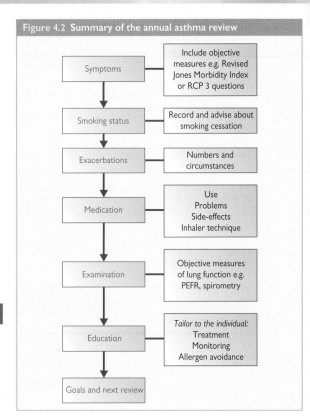

Figure 4.2 Summary of the annual asthma review

Symptoms → Include objective measures e.g. Revised Jones Morbidity Index or RCP 3 questions

Smoking status → Record and advise about smoking cessation

Exacerbations → Numbers and circumstances

Medication → Use / Problems / Side-effects / Inhaler technique

Examination → Objective measures of lung function e.g. PEFR, spirometry

Education → *Tailor to the individual:* Treatment / Monitoring / Allergen avoidance

Goals and next review

Further information

British Thoracic Society/SIGN: British guideline on the management of asthma (revised 2004) 🖳 www.sign.ac.uk

Cochrane: Accessed via 🖳 www.nelh.nhs.uk

- Gibson *et al.* Self-management education and regular practitioner review for adults with asthma (2002)
- Gøtzsche *et al.* House dust mite control measures for asthma (2004)
- Kilburn *et al.* Pet allergen control measures for allergic asthma in children and adults (2001)

GMS contract			
Asthma 1	The practice can produce a register of patients with asthma, excluding patients with asthma who have been prescribed no asthma-related drugs in the last 12 mo.	4 points	
Asthma 3	% of patients with asthma aged 14–19y. in whom there is a record of smoking status in the previous 15mo.	up to 6 points	40–80%
Asthma 6	% of patients with asthma who have had an asthma review in the last 15 mo. This should include: • Assessment of symptoms • Measurement of peak flow • Assessment of inhaler technique • Consideration of a personalised asthma plan	up to 20 points	40-70%
Smoking 1	% of patients with any/combination of: • coronary heart disease • stroke or TIA • hypertension • diabetes • COPD or asthma whose notes record smoking status in the previous 15 mo. Except those who have never smoked where smoking status need only be recorded once since diagnosis	up to 33 points	40-90%
Smoking 2	% of patients with any/combination of the conditions listed in 'smoking 1' who smoke whose notes contain a record that smoking cessation advice or referral to a specialist service, where available, has been offered within the previous 15 mo.	up to 35 points	40-90%
Records 22	% of patients aged >15y. whose notes record smoking status in the past 27 mo., except those who have never smoked where smoking status need be recorded only once.	up to 11 points	40-90%
Information 5	The practice supports smokers in stopping smoking by a strategy which includes providing literature and offering appropriate therapy.	2 points	
Medicines 12	A medication review is recorded in the notes in the preceding 15 mo. for all patients being prescribed repeat medicines.	8 points	Minimum 80%

Drug therapy: Use a stepwise approach (Figure 4.3). Start at the step most appropriate to the initial severity of symptoms. The aim is to achieve early control of the condition and then to ↓ treatment by stepping down.

> ⚠ **Exacerbations:** People still die of asthma – step up rapidly during exacerbations, step down slowly. A rescue course of prednisolone 30–40mg od for 1–2wk. may be needed at any step and any time.

Stepping down: Review and consider stepping down at intervals ≥3mo. Maintain on the lowest dose of inhaled steroid controlling symptoms. When reducing steroids, cut dose by 25-50% each time.

Selection of inhaler device:
- If possible use a metred dose inhaler (MDI).
- Inadequate technique may be mistaken for drug failure.
- Emphasize patients must inhale slowly and hold their breath for 10sec. after inhalation.
- Demonstrate inhaler technique before prescribing and check at follow-ups.
- Spacers or breath-activated devices are useful for patients who find activation difficult.
- Dry powder inhalers are an alternative.

114

GP Notes: Use of spacers with metred dose inhalers

Advantages of using a spacer:
- Allows more time for evaporation of propellant so a larger proportion of active drug is deposited in the lungs.
- There is no need to coordinate actuation with inhalation.
- Less oro-pharyngeal side-effects (e.g. thrush, hoarseness) occur with inhaled steroids if delivered via a spacer.

Choice of spacer: Large volumatic spacers are no longer manufactured. Medium-volume devices (e.g. aerochamber) are widely available, acceptable and portable.

Use of spacer devices: Inhale the drug from the spacer immediately after actuation as effect of the drugs is short-lived. Spacers should be washed and air-dried weekly to prevent build-up of electrostatic charge affecting drug delivery, and replaced every 6–12mo.

Advice for patients: Information and support for patients

Asthma UK ☎ 08457 01 02 03 🖥 www.asthma.org.uk

Further information
British Thoracic Society/SIGN British guideline on the management of asthma (revised 2004) 🖥 www.sign.ac.uk

Figure 4.3 Summary of stepwise management in adults

Step 5: Continuous or frequent use of oral steroids:
Use daily steroid tablet in lowest dose providing adequate control
Maintain high-dose inhaled steroid at 2000mcgm/d.*
Consider other treatments to minimise the use of steroid tablets
Refer patient for respiratory opinion

Step 4: Persistent poor control
Consider trials of:
-Increase inhaled steroid to 2000mcgm/d.*
-Addition of a 4th drug e.g. leukotriene receptor agonist, SR theophylline, β_2 agonist tablet

Step 3: Add-on threrapy
- Add inhaled long-acting β_2 agonist (LABA)
- Assess control of asthma:
- Good response to LABA – continue LABA
- Benefit from LABA but control still inadequate – continue LABA and ↑ inhaled steroid dose to 800mcgm/d.*
- No response to LABA – stop LABA and ↑ inhaled steroid dose to 800mcgm/d.* If control is still inadequate, institute trial of other therapies e.g. leukotriene receptor antagonists or SR theophylline

Step 2: Regular preventer therapy
Add inhaled steroid 200–800mcgm/d.*
400µg/d. is an appropriate starting point for most adults
Start at dose of steroid appropriate to severity of disease

Step 1: Mild intermittent asthma
Inhaled short-acting β_2 agonist as required

* Beclometasone dipropionate or equivalent

All doses given refer to beclometasone dipropionate (BDP) administered via metred dose inhaler. For other drugs/formulations adjust dose accordingly (see *BNF* Section 3).

Figure 4.3 is reproduced from the British guideline on the management of asthma (2004) with permission from SIGN/British Thoracic Society.

Drugs: BNF 3.1, 3.2 & 3.3

Short-acting β₂ agonists: *e.g. salbutamol, terbutaline.* Cause relaxation of bronchial smooth muscle. Safest, most effective β_2 agonists for use as quick relievers in asthma.
- Duration of action: ~3–5h. Oral preparations are less effective than inhaled preparations. Prescribe as 1–2 puffs prn unless shown to benefit from regular dosing.
- Warn patients to seek medical advice if usual dose does not relieve symptoms or relieves symptoms for <3h.
- Consider using a nebulizer if high doses are needed.
- Regular treatment with bronchodilators alone may be linked with worsening of asthma and asthma deaths. If asthmatic and using >1x/d. consider starting prophylaxis.
- Using ≥1 canister/mo. or >10–12 puffs/d. is a marker of poorly controlled asthma.

Inhaled corticosteroids: Most effective preventer for achieving overall treatment goals. Use regularly to obtain maximum benefit. Alleviation of symptoms occurs 3–7d. after initiation. Supply patients using high-dose inhalers with a 'steroid card'. May be beneficial even for patients with mild asthma. *Consider if:*
- Exacerbations of asthma in the last 2y.
- Using inhaled β_2 agonists >3x/wk.
- Symptomatic ≥3x/wk. or ≥1 night /wk.

Problems
- If the inhaled corticosteroid causes coughing, a short-acting β_2 agonist before use might help.
- Common unwanted effects are oral candidiasis (5%) and hoarseness – ↓ by use of a large-volume spacer or mouth washing after use.

Oral steroids: Often started at high dose (40–50mg od for ≥5d. or until necessary) to suppress disease process and control exacerbations of asthma, and stopped once symptoms are improved. Rarely used as maintenance therapy – use the minimum dose that controls disease. Prescribe as a single dose in the morning to ↓ circadian rhythm disturbance. Supply with a 'steroid card'.

Side-effects: Box 4.3

Withdrawal of steroids: Stop abruptly if the patient has received treatment for ≤3wk., is not included in the groups described below and is taking inhaled steroids. Withdraw gradually if the patient has:
- Recently had repeated steroid courses (particularly if taken for >3wk.)
- Taken a short course <1y. after stopping long-term therapy
- Other possible causes of adrenal suppression
- Been given repeat doses in the evening
- Received treatment with steroids for >3wk.

⓵ During corticosteroid withdrawal, ↓ dose rapidly to physiological levels (~ prednisolone 7.5mg od) – thereafter ↓ more slowly. Assess during withdrawal to ensure symptoms don't recur.

⚠ If poor control, check compliance and inhaler technique before altering medication.

Box 4.3 Side-effects of oral and high-dose inhaled steroids

- ↑ BP
- Osteoporosis ± fracture – long-term use or recurrent short courses – consider prophylaxis with a bisphosphonate
- Proximal muscle wasting
- Euphoria
- Paranoid states or depression – especially if past history of psychiatric disorder
- Peptic ulceration – ↑ risk if also taking NSAIDs. Soluble or enteric-coated (EC) versions may ↓ risk. Consider protecting gastric mucosa with a PPI or misoprostol – especially if taking a NSAID concurrently
- Suppression of clinical signs – may allow diseases e.g. septicaemia to reach advanced stage before being recognized
- Spread of infection e.g. chickenpox, oral thrush
- Hyperglycaemia in non-diabetic patients (consider weekly urine monitoring for glucose followed up by fasting blood glucose if positive) and worsening of diabetic control in diabetic patients
- Cushing's syndrome – moon face, striae and acne
- Adrenal atrophy – can persist for years after stopping long-term steroids – illness or surgical emergencies may require steroid supplements
- Frail skin which bruises easily
- Na^+ and water retention; K^+ loss

117

GP Notes: Steroid cards

Should be carried at all times by patients on oral or high doses of inhaled steroids. The card:
- Informs other practitioners your patient is on steroids *and*
- Gives the patient advice on use of steroids and risk of infection.

Obtaining steroid cards
- England and Wales: Department of Health ☎ 08701 555 455
- Scotland: Banner Business Supplies ☎ 01506 448 440

Add-on therapy: Before initiating a new drug, check compliance, inhaler technique and eliminate trigger factors.

Longer-acting β$_2$ agonists (LABA): e.g. salmeterol, formoterol. Inhaled preparations (e.g. salmeterol 50–100mcgm bd) improve lung function/symptoms. Slow-release tablets have similar effect but side-effects are greater. Don't use without inhaled steroids. Particularly useful for night-time asthma. Usual duration of action is ~12h. Do not use for relief of acute attacks.

Theophylline

- Improves lung function and symptoms.
- Narrow therapeutic range – side-effects and toxicity are common. Plasma theophylline concentration for optimum response is 10–20mg/l (55–110micromol/l).
- Side-effects include cardiovascular symptoms (palpitations/ tachycardia/arrhythmia), GI disturbance and CNS symptoms (headache, hyperactivity, insomnia, convulsions).

⚠ Prescribe slow-release theophylline preparations by brand name (and NOT genericallly) as bioavailability varies between brands. Available preparations include:
- Slo-phyllin 175–350mg bd
- Nuelin SA 250–500mg bd
- Uniphyllin Continus 400mg daily – in bd divided doses or rarely single dose – increased as needed to 800mg daily
- Phyllocontin Continus 225mg bd increased after 1wk. to 450mg bd.

Leukotriene receptor antagonists: e.g. montelukast (10mg od in the evening), zafirlukast (20mg bd). Provide improvement in symptoms and lung function, and ↓ exacerbations.

Sodium cromoglycate and nedocromil sodium: Some evidence of benefit in adults (nedocromil sodium > sodium cromoglycate).

Complementary and alternative therapies: Table 4.4

Home nebulizer therapy: In England and Wales nebulizers are not available via the NHS (but are free of VAT). Some nebulizers are available in Scotland on form GP10A. Nebulizers convert a solution of drug into an aerosol for inhalation. They are used to deliver a higher dosage of drug than is usual with inhalers over a short period of time (5–10min.).

List of available devices: BNF 3.1.5

Indications

- Acute exacerbations ± regular treatment of asthma
- Antibiotic treatment – for patients with chronic purulent infection e.g. CF, bronchiectasis, prophylaxis and treatment of pneumocystis pneumonia with pentamidine in patients with AIDS
- Palliative care – palliation of breathlessness and cough e.g. bronchodilators, lignocaine or bupivacaine for dry, persistent cough

Table 4.4 Evidence for use of complementary therapies in asthma

Evidence	Therapy	
Inconclusive but some evidence of benefit	• Acupuncture[C] • Physical training[C] • Immunotherapy[C] – only in specialized clinics	• Breathing exercises[C] • Herbal medicine[S]
Insufficient evidence	• Massage[C] • Relaxation therapies[S]	• Homeopathy[C]
No benefit	• Chiropractic[C]	• Fish oil supplements[C]

GP Notes: Use of home nebulizers for patients with asthma/COPD

Before suggesting long-term use:
• Review diagnosis
• Review technique using hand-held device e.g. MDI ± spacer
• Review compliance with medication
• Try ↑ dose of bronchodilator via a hand-held device for at least 2wk.
• Perform a 2wk. trial of nebulizer therapy and monitor therapeutic effect (e.g. with PEFR in asthma, or dyspnoea score with COPD).

Provide clear instructions on the use of the nebulizer, monitoring and when to seek help.

ⓘ All patients with home nebulizers should be followed up regularly.

Advice for patients: Information and support for patients

Asthma UK ☎ 08457 01 02 03 🖥 www.asthma.org.uk

Further information

British Thoracic Society Current best practice for nebuliser treatment *Thorax* (1997) **52**(Suppl 2): S4–24
🖥 www.brit-thoracic.org.uk
Cochrane: Accessed via 🖥 www.nelh.nhs.uk
• Ram et al. Physical training for asthma (2005)
• McCarney et al. Acupuncture for chronic asthma (2003)
• Dennis & Cates Alexander technique for chronic asthma (2000)
• Abramson et al. Allergen immunotherapy for asthma (2003)
• Holloway & Ram Breathing exercises for asthma (2004)
• Thien et al. Dietary marine fatty acids (fish oil) for asthma in adults and children (2002)
• McCarney et al. Homeopathy for chronic asthma (2004)
• Hondras et al. Manual therapy for asthma (2005)
Thorax:
• Huntley & Ernst Herbal medicines for asthma: a systematic review (2000) **55**(11): 925–9
• Huntley et al. Relaxation therapies for asthma: a systematic review (2002) **57**(2): 127–31

Immunization: All asthmatics should be offered:
- Influenza vaccination each year[£]
- Pneumococcal vaccination. Give once. Booster doses are not needed except for patients with asplenia or nephrotic syndrome – when give a booster after 5–10y.

Psychosocial factors: Depression, anxiety and denial of disease are associated strongly with asthma deaths. Other associations with asthma severity include life crises, family conflict, social isolation, shame, anger and high-risk lifestyles e.g. smoking and alcohol abuse. When asthma proves difficult to control on usually effective therapy, find out about any family, psychological or social problems which may be interfering with effective management.

Referral: Consider referral to a respiratory or general physician if:
- Stridor E
- Chest pain E
- Non-resolving pneumonia E/U
- Unilateral or fixed wheeze U
- Weight loss U
- Persistent shortness of breath/symptoms despite treatment U/S
- Persistent cough ± sputum production U/S/R
- Abnormal CXR U/S/R
- Unexpected clinical findings (e.g. clubbing, cyanosis) U/S/R
- Spirometry or PEFR does not fit the clinical picture S/R
- Suspected occupational asthma R.

E=Emergency admission; U=Urgent; S=Soon; R=Routine

❶ This is only a rough guide, urgency of referral depends on clinical state.

Management of children <12y.: 📖 pp.76–83

Asthma in pregnancy: Affects ≈5% of pregnant women.
- Generally improves with pregnancy, especially into the 3rd trimester.
- In most cases treat asthma as usual – there is no evidence that any of the drugs commonly used to treat asthma cause birth defects, problems in pregnancy or with breast feeding. ❶ Leukotriene receptor antagonists have limited safety data in pregnancy – seek specialist advice.
- Women with very badly controlled asthma are more at risk of early labour and intrauterine growth retardation.
- Women on oral steroids may require IV steroids to cover labour.
- Avoid syntometrine for 3rd stage of labour as it contains ergometrine which can cause a severe attack.
- There is a tendency to worsening of asthma after delivery.

Occupational asthma: 📖 p.182

Further information

British Thoracic Society/SIGN British guideline on the management of asthma (revised 2004) 🖥 www.sign.ac.uk
Clinical evidence: Dennis *et al.* Asthma (2004). Accessed via 🖥 www.nelh.nhs.uk

GMS contract

Influenza and pneumococcal vaccination may be offered by GMS practices as a directed enhanced service – 📖 p.246

Chronic obstructive pulmonary disease

Chronic obstructive pulmonary disease (COPD) is a slowly progressive disorder characterized by airflow obstruction. It affects ~16% of the population in the 40–68y. age group (♂>♀) and is responsible for ~5% of deaths.

Causes
- Cigarette smoking
- Genetic – bronchial hyper-responsiveness; α_1-antitrypsin deficiency
- Race – Chinese & Afro-Caribbeans have ↓ susceptibility
- Nutritional – poor diet and low birthweight are risk factors

Presentation: Affects different patients in different ways. Diagnosis is suggested by a combination of history, signs and baseline spirometry.

History: Consider diagnosis in any patient >35y. with a risk factor for COPD (generally smoking) and ≥1 of:
- Shortness of breath on exertion – use an objective measure e.g. MRC dyspnoea scale (Table 4.6) to grade breathlessness
- Chronic cough
- Regular sputum production
- Frequent winter 'bronchitis'
- Wheeze.

If a diagnosis of COPD is suspected also ask about:
- Weight ↓
- Effort intolerance
- Waking at night
- Ankle swelling
- Fatigue
- Occupational hazards.

⚠ Chest pain or haemoptysis are uncommon in COPD – if present consider an alternative diagnosis.

Signs: May be none. Possible signs:
- Hyperinflated chest ± poor chest expansion on inspiration
- ↓ crico-sternal distance
- Hyper-resonant chest with ↓ cardiac dullness on percussion
- Use of accessory muscles
- Paradoxical movement of lower ribs
- Tachypnoea
- Wheeze or quiet breath sounds
- Pursing of lips on expiration (purse-lip breathing)
- Peripheral oedema
- Cyanosis
- ↑ JVP
- Cachexia.

Table 4.5 Comparison of COPD and asthma

Symptom	COPD	Asthma
Symptoms <35y.	Rare	Common
Smoking history	Nearly all	Maybe
Breathlessness	Persistent and progressive. Poor response to inhaled therapy – if good reconsider diagnosis	Variable throughout the day and from day to day. Good response to inhaled therapy typical
Chronic productive cough	Common	Uncommon
Waking at night with cough/wheeze	Uncommon	Common

Table 4.6 MRC dyspnoea scale

Grade	Degree of breathlessness related to physical activity
1	Not troubled by breathlessness except on strenuous exercise
2	Short of breath when hurrying or walking up a slight hill
3	Walks slower than contemporaries on level ground because of breathlessness or has to stop for breath when walking at own pace
4	Stops for breath after walking about 100m or after a few minutes on level ground
5	Too breathless to leave the house or breathless on dressing/undressing

GP Notes: Patients with severe COPD

Tend to fall into one of 2 categories:

Blue bloaters: Severe COPD +
- Cyanosis ('blue') due to CO_2 retention *and*
- Right heart failure ('bloater')
- Cough and sputum production

❶ Patients don't always appear breathless (compare with pink puffers)

Pink puffers: Severe COPD +
- Thin
- No cyanosis ('pink')
- Breathless ('puffer') – working hard to maintain sufficient oxygenation to avoid cyanosis

Table 4.6 is reproduced with permission from the MRC.

Tests

Spirometry: Predicts prognosis but not disability/quality of life – Figure 4.4.
A diagnosis of airflow obstruction can be made if:
- FEV_1/FVC <0.7 (<70%) *and*
- FEV_1 <70% predicted (Quality and Outcomes Framework criterion) or <80% predicted (British Thoracic Society guidelines) *and*
- <15% response to a reversibility test.
- Reversibility testing may be confusing but is currently required for the Quality and Outcomes Framework targets:
- >400ml ↑ in FEV_1 following trial of bronchodilator or prednisolone (30mg od for 2 wk.) suggests asthma
- Clinically significant COPD is *not* present if FEV_1 and FEV_1/FVC return to normal after drug therapy.

PEFR
- Patients with COPD have little variability in PEFR.
- Serial home PEFR measurements can help distinguish between asthma and COPD.
- PEFR may underestimate severity of airflow limitation and a normal PEFR does not exclude airflow obstruction.

CXR: Indicated to exclude other diagnoses e.g. lung cancer.

FBC: To identify polycythaemia $2°$ to chronic lung disease or anaemia which might be making symptoms worse.

Body mass index: If obese, weight loss may increase exercise tolerance. Weight loss and cachexia may be a sign of severe disease – consider nutritional supplements.

Other investigations: Only if indicated clinically:
- α_1-antitrypsin – if early-onset COPD or family history
- ECG/echo – if cor pulmonale suspected
- Sputum culture – if persistent purulent sputum.

Differential diagnosis
- Asthma
- Bronchiectasis
- Congestive cardiac failure (sometimes coexists)
- Lung cancer

GMS contract

COPD 1	The practice can produce a register of patients with COPD	3 points	
COPD 9	% of all patients with COPD in whom diagnosis has been confirmed by spirometry including reversibility testing	up to 10 points	40–80%

⚠ Patients should not be on the asthma AND COPD register. If the patient was previously on the asthma register but now has COPD, code as inactive on asthma register.

Table 4.7 Severity of COPD and expected clinical picture

Severity	Clinical state	Spirometry
Mild	Cough but little or no breathlessness. No abnormal signs. No ↑ use of services.	FEV_1 50–80% predicted
Moderate	Breathlessness, wheeze on exertion, cough ± sputum and some abnormal signs. Usually known to GP – intermittent complaints.	FEV_1 30–49% predicted
Severe	SOBOE. Marked wheeze and cough. Usually other signs too. Likely to be known to GP and hospital consultant with frequent problems/admissions.	FEV_1 <30% predicted

Advice for patients: Information and support for patients

British Lung Foundation ☎ 08458 50 50 20
🖥 www.lunguk.org

Figure 4.4 Flow volume curve for a patient with COPD

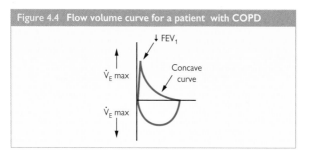

Management of COPD

Aims of treatment
- To minimize symptoms and impact on lifestyle (e.g. absence from work; limitations to physical ability)
- To prevent severe attacks/exacerbations

Management of acute exacerbation of COPD: 📖 p.134

GP services: Ideally routine care for patients with COPD should be carried out in a specialized clinic. Doctors and nurses involved in COPD clinics need appropriate training with regular updates. Practices should keep a COPD register of affected patients to ensure adequate follow-up and allow audit[L].

Self-management: All patients/carers should receive:
- *Self-management education:* Brief, simple education linked to patient goals is most likely to be successful. Include information about: nature of disease, nature of the treatment and how to use it, self-monitoring/self-assessment, recognition of acute exacerbations, allergen/trigger avoidance, patient's own goals of treatment.
- *Written action plan:* Focus on individual needs. Include information about features which indicate when COPD is worsening and what to do under those circumstances. Action plans help patients recognize exacerbations and start medication sooner. It is not clear whether this translates into ↓ morbidity/mortality/health costs[C].

Reviews and monitoring[L]:
Frequency depends on needs. Aim to review all patients with COPD at least annually (Figure 4.5) and more frequently if severe COPD (every 6mo.) and/or altering treatment.

- Check symptoms since last seen. Use objective measures e.g. the MRC dyspnoea scale (Table 4.6, 📖 p.123).
- Record smoking status of patients with COPD – advise smokers to stop[L].
- Record any exacerbations/change in symptoms since last seen.
- Record body mass index.
- Check medication[L] – use, concordance (prescription count), inhaler technique[L], problems, side-effects.
- Influenza and pneumococcal vaccination should be offered to all patients with COPD[L].
- Review objective measures of lung function e.g. spirometry, oxygen saturation (if available) at review[L]. Compare with previous values and values at diagnosis.
- Review mood – depression is common in patients with severe COPD.
- Review the need for referral for specialist care (📖 p.132).
- Address any problems or queries and educate about COPD.
- Check all benefits the patient/carer is eligible for have been applied for and patient and carer are coping at home. Consider referral for OT review/social services assessment if appropriate.
- Agree management goals and date for further review.

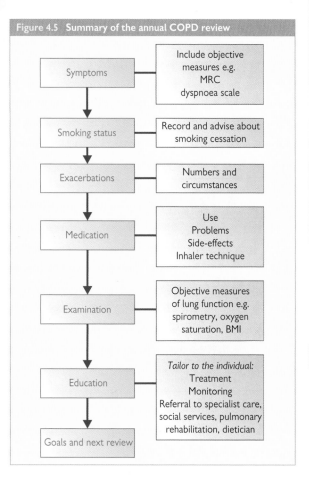

Figure 4.5 Summary of the annual COPD review

Symptoms — Include objective measures e.g. MRC dyspnoea scale

Smoking status — Record and advise about smoking cessation

Exacerbations — Numbers and circumstances

Medication — Use / Problems / Side-effects / Inhaler technique

Examination — Objective measures of lung function e.g. spirometry, oxygen saturation, BMI

Education — Tailor to the individual: Treatment / Monitoring / Referral to specialist care, social services, pulmonary rehabilitation, dietician

Goals and next review

Further information
British Thoracic Society/SIGN: British guideline on the management of asthma (revised 2004) www.sign.ac.uk
Cochrane: Turnock et al. Action plans for chronic obstructive pulmonary disease (2005). Accessed via www.nelh.nhs.uk

GMS contract			
COPD 1	The practice can produce a register of patients with COPD	3 points	
COPD 8	% of COPD patients who have had influenza vaccine in the preceding 1st September - 31st March	up to 6 points	40-85%
COPD 10	% of COPD patients with a record of FEV1 in the previous 15mo.	up to 7 points	40-70%
COPD 11	% of patients with COPD receiving inhaled treatment in whom there is a record that inhaler technique has been checked in the previous 15mo.	up to 7 points	40-90%
Smoking 1	% of patients with any/combination of: • coronary heart disease • stroke or TIA • hypertension • diabetes • COPD or asthma whose notes record smoking status in the previous 15 mo. Except those who have never smoked where smoking status need only be recorded once since diagnosis	up to 33 points	40-90%
Smoking 2	% of patients with any/combination of the conditions listed in 'smoking 1' who smoke whose notes contain a record that smoking cessation advice or referral to a specialist service, where available, has been offered within the previous 15 mo.	up to 35 points	40-90%
Records 22	% of patients aged >15y. whose notes record smoking status in the past 27 mo., except those who have never smoked where smoking status need be recorded only once.	up to 11 points	40-90%
Information 5	The practice supports smokers in stopping smoking by a strategy which includes providing literature and offering appropriate therapy.	2 points	
Medicines 12	A medication review is recorded in the notes in the preceding 15 mo. for all patients being prescribed repeat medicines.	8 points	Minimum 80%

Advice for patients: Information and support for patients

British Lung Foundation ☎ 08458 50 50 20
🖥 www.lunguk.org

Advice for patients: Frequently asked questions about COPD

What is COPD?
COPD (chronic obstructive pulmonary disease) is a term which covers the conditions chronic bronchitis (inflammation of the large airways) and emphysema (damage to the small airways and airsacs). These 2 conditions often occur together and are treated the same way. COPD mainly affects people over 40 years of age and is very common in the UK. COPD has similar symptoms to asthma but differs from asthma because the changes are permanent and not completely reversible with medicine. Asthma and COPD can occur together in the same person.

What causes COPD?
• Smoking is the cause of COPD in most cases.

What are the symptoms of COPD?
• Cough with phlegm – usually the first symptom to develop.
• Breathlessness and wheeze – usually only on exercise e.g. climbing stairs at first.
• Chest infections are more common. Cough and breathing difficulties become worse and phlegm turns green or yellow.

❶ COPD is progressive so symptoms gradually get worse with time.

How is the diagnosis made?
Your symptoms will suggest the diagnosis. The doctor may examine you to see if you have any other features of COPD. Usually the test which confirms diagnosis is a lung test called spirometry. You will be asked to blow into a special machine. It measures how well your lungs are functioning. Other tests might also be done to exclude other conditions.

What can I do to help myself?
• Give up smoking: smoking increases symptoms of COPD and makes the lungs deteriorate faster. Stopping smoking will help your lungs more than anything else. Cigarette smoke from other people in your home can also make symptoms worse so encourage them to stop too – or at least ask them not to smoke in your home.
• Lose weight: this improves symptoms of COPD if you are over-weight.
• Exercise: lack of exercise makes breathing worse. Keep your exercise levels up and try to stay as fit as you can.

What is the treatment for COPD?
• Symptoms usually become worse if you continue to smoke. Symptoms are likely to stabilize if you stop smoking.
• Treatment with inhalers often eases symptoms, but no treatment can reverse the damage to the airways.
• A flare-up of symptoms, often during a chest infection, may be helped by a short course of steroid tablets and/or antibiotics.
• Immunization against flu and pneumococcal infection is a good idea to prevent chest infections.

Non-drug therapy

- *Smoking cessation[E]:* Most important way to improve outcome (Figure 4.6). Encourage at every opportunity – 🕮 p.136.
- *Vaccination:* All patients with COPD should have influenza and pneumococcal vaccination[E].
- *Exercise:* Lack of exercise ↓ FEV$_1$. Encourage exercise either through a formal exercise prescription scheme or by increasing level of activity attached to everyday activities (e.g. advise walking to work). Pulmonary rehabilitation is aimed at patients who are functionally disabled by COPD. Pulmonary rehabilitation ↓ dyspnoea and fatigue and ↑ exercise capacity and sense of control. Particularly suitable for patients with moderate/severe COPD and/or disabling symptoms. Refer via respiratory physicians if available locally[C].
- *Nutrition:* Weight ↓ in obese patients improves exercise tolerance. In more advanced disease, patients may need dietary advice ± supplements to maintain weight.

Drug therapy: Document effects of each drug treatment on symptoms, quality of life and lung function as tried. In mild cases, smoking cessation may be the only treatment needed. Treat if breathless with a short-acting bronchodilator e.g. salbutamol 1–2 puffs prn ± long-acting bronchodilator ± inhaled steroid depending on FEV$_1$, symptom control and frequency of exacerbations – Figure 4.7.

- If possible use a metred dose inhaler (MDI). Spacers or breath-activated devices are useful for patients who find activation difficult. Dry powder inhalers are an alternative.
- Inadequate technique may be mistaken for drug failure.
- Emphasize patients must inhale slowly and hold breath for 10sec. after inhalation.
- Demonstrate inhaler technique before prescribing and check at each review.

Other drugs

- *Tiotropium* is a long-acting anticholinergic bronchodilator. It ↓ COPD exacerbations and hospitalizations, improves quality of life and slows decline of FEV$_1$. Its place in management is not yet established as there is little evidence about how it compares to standard treatments[C].
- *Antibiotics* have a role in treatment of acute exacerbations of COPD. There is no evidence that they are helpful as prophylaxis.
- *Phosphodiesterase type 4 inhibitors* (e.g. cilomilast). At present there is insufficient evidence of efficacy to recommend routine use.
- *Oral steroids* are effective for treatment of acute exacerbations[C] (🕮 p.134). There is no evidence to support long-term use of oral steroids at doses <10–15mg prednisolone od. Doses ≥30mg od improve lung function over a short period but use is limited by side-effects (🕮 p.117). Avoid long-term oral steroids if possible.

Anxiety and depression: Anxiety and depression are common amongst patients with COPD. It can be difficult to decide if patients are depressed as some of the symptoms of severe COPD overlap with symptoms of depression. Offer all patients with COPD support and, if in doubt, a trial of antidepressants is worthwhile.

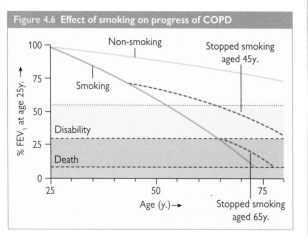

Figure 4.6 **Effect of smoking on progress of COPD**

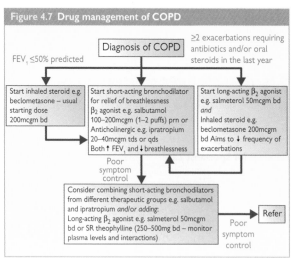

Figure 4.7 **Drug management of COPD**

Figure 4.6 is reproduced in modified format from Fletcher & Peto, *BMJ* (1977) 1: 1645–8.

Home nebulizer therapy: In England and Wales nebulizers are not available via the NHS (but are free of VAT). Some nebulizers are available in Scotland on form GP10A. Nebulizers convert a solution of drug into an aerosol for inhalation. They are used to deliver a higher dosage of drug than is usual with inhalers over a short period of time (5–10min.).

List of available devices: BNF 3.1.5

Indications: Consider if the patient is taking maximum inhaler therapy but still has distressing or disabling breathlessness. Arrange training for patient or carer. Continue use *only* if there is improvement in symptoms, activities, exercise capacity or lung function.

❶ Supply a mouthpiece rather than face mask if delivering anticholinergics via a nebulizer.

Long-term oxygen therapy (LTOT): *Only* prescribe after evaluation by a respiratory physician. Refer patients with:

- Severe airflow obstruction ($FEV_1 < 30\%$ – consider if 30–49%)
- Cyanosis
- Polycythaemia
- Peripheral oedema
- ↑JVP
- Hypoxaemia (oxygen saturation ≤92% breathing air)

Treatment for >15h./d. ↑ survival and quality of life for patients with severe hypoxaemia only[C]. Ambulatory oxygen therapy can ↑ exercise tolerance in some patients[C].

❶ Always warn patients about the fire risks of having pure oxygen in their home.

132

O_2 cylinders and associated equipment: O_2 concentrators are more economical for LTOT. Prescribe on FP10. Specify amount of O_2 required (h./d.) and flow rate. Arrangements for supply vary – see *BNF Section 3.6.* Supply back-up cylinders in case of breakdown or power cut.

Referral for specialist care

- Haemoptysis U
- Rapid decline in FEV_1 U/S
- Uncertain diagnosis U/S/R
- Severe COPD U/S/R
- Cor pulmonale S
- Frequent infections S/R
- Age <40y. R
- α_1-antitrypsin deficiency R
- Assessment for:
  - LTOT (see above) R
  - Long-term oral steroids R
  - withdrawal of long-term steroids R
  - long-term nebulizer therapy R
  - pulmonary rehabilitation R
  - surgery e.g. lung transplant R.

U=Urgent; S=Soon; R=Routine

❶ This is only a rough guide, urgency of referral depends on clinical state.

GP Notes: Use of home nebulizers for patients with asthma/ COPD

Before suggesting long-term use:
• Review diagnosis
• Review technique using hand-held device e.g. MDI ± spacer
• Review compliance with medication
• Try ↑ dose of bronchodilator via a hand-held device for at least 2wk.
• Perform a 2wk. trial of nebulizer therapy and monitor therapeutic effect (e.g. with PEFR in asthma, or dyspnoea score with COPD).
Provide clear instructions on the use of the nebulizer, monitoring and when to seek help.

❶ All patients with home nebulizers should be followed up regularly.

Advice for patients: Information and support for patients

British Lung Foundation ☎ 08458 50 50 20 🖥 www.lunguk.org

Further information

RCP/NICE National clinical guideline on management of chronic obstructive pulmonary disease in adults in primary and secondary care. *Thorax* (2004) **59**(Suppl 1): S1–232

Cochrane Accessed via 🖥 www.nelh.nhs.uk
• Lacasse *et al.* Pulmonary rehabilitation for chronic obstructive pulmonary disease (2001)
• Barr *et al.* Tiotropium for stable chronic obstructive pulmonary disease (2005)
• Walters *et al.* Oral corticosteroids for stable chronic obstructive pulmonary disease (2005)
• Wood-Baker *et al.* Systemic corticosteroids for acute exacerbations of chronic obstructive pulmonary disease (2005)
• Cranston *et al.* Domiciliary oxygen for chronic obstructive pulmonary disease (2005)
• Bradley & O'Neill Short-term ambulatory oxygen for chronic obstructive pulmonary disease (2005)

Acute exacerbations of COPD

Presentation: Worsening of previous stable condition.

Features: ≥1 of:
- ↑ dyspnoea – marked dyspnoea, tachypnoea (>25 breaths/min.), use of accessory muscles at rest and purse-lip breathing are signs of severe exacerbation
- ↓ exercise tolerance – marked ↓ in activities of daily living is a sign of severe exacerbation
- ↑ fatigue
- ↑ fluid retention – new-onset oedema is a sign of severe exacerbation
- ↑ wheeze
- Chest tightness
- ↑ cough
- ↑ sputum purulence
- ↑ sputum volume
- Upper airways symptoms e.g. colds, sore throats
- New-onset cyanosis – severe exacerbation
- Acute confusion – severe exacerbation.

🛈 Fever and chest pain are uncommon presenting features – consider alternative diagnosis.

Causes of exacerbations: 30% have no identifiable cause.
- *Infections:* Viral upper and lower respiratory tract infections e.g. common cold, influenza, bacterial lower respiratory tract infections.
- *Pollutants* e.g. nitrous oxide, sulphur dioxide, ozone.

Differential diagnosis
- Pneumonia
- LVF/pulmonary oedema
- Lung cancer
- Pleural effusion
- Recurrent aspiration
- Pneumothorax
- PE
- Upper airway obstruction

Investigations
- *Pulse oximetry:* If available can be used as a measure of severity (saturation ≤92% breathing air suggests hypoxaemia – consider admission) and to monitor progress.
- *CXR:* Consider if diagnostic doubt and/or to exclude other causes of symptoms.
- *Sputum culture:* Not recommended routinely in the community[G].

Management: Decide whether to treat at home or admit to hospital – Table 4.8.

Home treatment of acute exacerbations
- *Add or ↑ bronchodilators:* Consider if inhaler device and technique are appropriate.
- *Start antibiotics:* Use broad-spectrum antibiotic e.g. erythromycin 250–500mg qds if sputum becomes more purulent *or* clinical signs of pneumonia *or* consolidation on CXR.

- *Oral corticosteroids:* Start early in the course of the exacerbation if ↑ breathlessness which interferes with daily activities. Dosage – 30mg/d. of prednisolone for 1–2wk. Consider osteoporosis prophylaxis with a bisphosphonate if frequent courses are required.

Follow-up

- Reassess as necessary. If the patient deteriorates reconsider the need for hospital admission (above). If not fully improved within 2wk. consider CXR and hospital referral.
- Reassess patients who have been admitted 4–6wk. after discharge. Assess their ability to cope at home. ~ 1:3 are readmitted within 3mo.
- Reassess inhaler technique and understanding of treatment regime.
- In severe cases, reassess the need for LTOT and/or home nebulizer.
- Check FEV_1.
- Emphasize the potential benefit of lifestyle modification – smoking cessation, exercise, weight loss if obese.
- Arrange ongoing regular follow-up.

Further information

RCP/NICE National clinical guideline on management of chronic obstructive pulmonary disease in adults in primary and secondary care. *Thorax* (2004) **59**(Suppl 1): S1–232

Table 4.8 Deciding whether to treat acute exacerbations at home or in hospital. (The more features in the 'treat in hospital' column, the more likely the need for admission)

	Treat at home	Treat in hospital*
Ability to cope at home	Yes	No
Breathlessness	Mild	Severe
General condition	Good	Poor – deteriorating
Level of activity	Good	Poor/confined to bed
Cyanosis	No	Yes
Worsening peripheral oedema	No	Yes
Level of consciousness	Normal	Impaired
Already receiving LTOT	No	Yes
Social circumstances	Good	Living alone/not coping
Acute confusion	No	Yes
Rapid rate of onset	No	Yes
Significant co-morbidity (e.g. cardiac disease, IDDM)	No	Yes
Changes on CXR (if available)	No	Present

*Hospital-at-home schemes and assisted discharge schemes are a suitable alternative.

Smoking

Facts and figures
- In the UK, 12 million adults (28% ♂; 26% ♀) smoke cigarettes and a further 3 million smoke pipes or cigars.
- Prevalence is highest in the 20–24y. old age group.
- 1% school children are smokers when they enter secondary school; by 15y., 22% are smoking.
- 82% of smokers start as teenagers.
- Government targets aim to ↓ smoking to ≤24% by 2010, and ↓ smoking amongst children to ≤9% by 2010.
- Surveys of smokers show 70% want to stop and 30% intend to give up in <1y., but only ~2%/y. give up permanently.

Risks of smoking: Smoking is the greatest single cause of illness and premature death in the UK. ½ all regular smokers will eventually die as a result of smoking – 120,000 people/y.

Tobacco smoking is associated with ↑ risk of
- *Cancers:* Lung (>90% are smokers), lip, mouth, stomach, colon, bladder. ~30% *ALL* cancer deaths are caused by smoking
- *Cardiovascular disease:* Arteriosclerosis, coronary heart disease, stroke, peripheral vascular disease
- *DM*
- *Chronic lung disease:* COPD, recurrent chest infection, exacerbation of asthma
- *Dyspepsia and/or gastric ulcers*
- *Thrombosis* (especially if also on the COC pill)
- *Osteoporosis*
- *Problems in pregnancy:* Pre-eclampsia, intra-uterine growth retardation, pre-term delivery, neonatal & late fetal death

Passive smoking is associated with:
- ↑ risk of coronary heart disease & lung cancer (↑ by 25%)
- ↑ risk of cot death, bronchitis and otitis media in children

Nicotine withdrawal symptoms
- Urges to smoke (70%)
- ↑ appetite (70% – average 3–4kg weight gain)
- Depression (60%)
- Restlessness (60%)
- Poor concentration (60%)
- Irritability/aggression (50%)
- Night-time awakenings (25%)
- Light-headedness (10% – usually 1st few days after quitting)

Helping people to stop smoking[£]: Advice from a GP about smoking cessation results in 2% of smokers stopping – 5% if advice is repeated[CE]. Strong motivation (often 2° to an episode of poor health directly related to smoking e.g. MI) is a vital factor.

Smoking: primary prevention

Records 22	% of patients aged >15y. whose notes record smoking status in the past 27 mo., except those who have never smoked where smoking status need be recorded only once.	up to 11 points	40-90%
Information 5	The practice supports smokers in stopping smoking by a strategy which includes providing literature and offering appropriate therapy.	2 points	

Smoking: secondary prevention

Asthma 3	% of patients with asthma aged 14-19y. in whom there is a record of smoking status in the previous 15 mo.	up to 6 points	40-80%
Smoking 1	% of patients with any/combination of: • coronary heart disease • stroke or TIA • hypertension • diabetes • COPD or asthma whose notes record smoking status in the previous 15 mo. Except those who have never smoked where smoking status need only be recorded once since diagnosis	up to 33 points	40-90%
Smoking 2	% of patients with any/combination of the conditions listed in 'smoking 1' who smoke whose notes contain a record that smoking cessation advice or referral to a specialist service, where available, has been offered within the previous 15 mo.	up to 35 points	40-90%

137

Advice for patients:

Useful contacts for patients

Action on Smoking and Health (ASH) ☎ 020 7739 5902
🖳 www.ash.org.uk
NHS smoking helpline ☎ 0800 169 0 169; pregnancy smoking
helpline: ☎ 0800 169 9 169 🖳 www.givingupsmoking.co.uk
Quit helpline ☎ 0800 00 22 00 🖳 www.quit.org.uk

Aids to smoking cessation: *BNF 4.10*

Nicotine replacement therapy (NRT)
- ↑ the chance of stopping ~1½ x[N].
- All preparations are equally effective[C] and available on NHS prescription.
- Start with higher doses for patients highly dependent.
- Continue treatment for 3mo., tailing off dose gradually over 2wk. before stopping (except gum which can be stopped abruptly).
- Several preparations are now licensed for use in pregnancy if unable to stop without NRT.
- Contraindicated immediately post MI, stroke or TIA, and for patients with arrhythmia.

Bupropion (Zyban™)
- Smokers (>18y.) start taking the tablets 1–2wk. before their intended quit day (150mg od for 3d. then 150mg bd for 7–9wk.).
- Effective treatment[C] which ↑ cessation rate >2x[N].
- *Contraindications:* epilepsy or ↑ risk of seizures, eating disorder, bipolar disorder, pregnancy/breast-feeding.

Alternative therapies: There is some evidence hypnotherapy is helpful in some cases[C].

Support: In many areas 'smoke stop' services are provided by local PCOs. These programmes vary from area to area but generally consist of a combination of group education, counselling and support ± individual support in combination with nicotine replacement or bupropion. There is very little evidence this type of support increases smoking cessation rates over and above rates achieved using medication alone[C].

138

Further information
Clinical evidence: Thorogood *et al.* Cardiovascular disorders: changing behaviour (2003). Accessed via 🖥 www.nelh.nhs.uk
NICE 🖥 www.nice.org.uk
- Smoking cessation: brief interventions and referral for smoking cessation in primary care and other settings (2006)
- Nicotine replacement and buprapion for smoking cessation (2002)
Cochrane: Accessed via 🖥 www.nelh.nhs.uk
- Stead & Lancaster Group behaviour therapy programmes for smoking cessation (2005)
- Hughes *et al.* Antidepressants for smoking cessation (2004)
- Silagy *et al.* Nicotine replacement for smoking cessation (2004)
- Abbot *et al.* Hypnotherapy for smoking cessation (1998)
BMJ Russell MAH Effect of GPs' advice against smoking (1979) **2**: 231–5
Thorax Smoking cessation guidelines for health professionals: an update (2000) **55**: 987–90 🖥 thorax.bmjjournals.com

Figure 4.8 Management plan for smokers in surgery

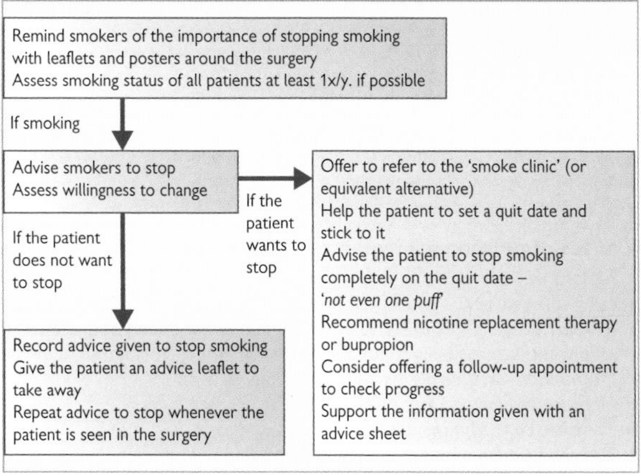

Remind smokers of the importance of stopping smoking with leaflets and posters around the surgery
Assess smoking status of all patients at least 1x/y. if possible

If smoking

Advise smokers to stop
Assess willingness to change

If the patient does not want to stop

If the patient wants to stop

Record advice given to stop smoking
Give the patient an advice leaflet to take away
Repeat advice to stop whenever the patient is seen in the surgery

Offer to refer to the 'smoke clinic' (or equivalent alternative)
Help the patient to set a quit date and stick to it
Advise the patient to stop smoking completely on the quit date –
'*not even one puff*'
Recommend nicotine replacement therapy or bupropion
Consider offering a follow-up appointment to check progress
Support the information given with an advice sheet

GP Notes:

⚠ Prescribe *only* for smokers who commit to target stop date. Initially prescribe only enough to last 2wk. after the target stop date i.e. 2wk. nicotine replacement therapy or 3–4wk. bupropion. Only offer a 2nd prescription if the smoker demonstrates continuing commitment to stop smoking.

❶ If unsuccessful the NHS will not fund another attempt for ≥6mo.

Pulmonary hypertension and cor pulmonale

Normal pulmonary arterial pressure is $<1/5$ of that in the systemic circulation. Pulmonary hypertension occurs by one of 3 mechanisms:
- High pulmonary blood flow (e.g. left → right shunt)
- ↑ pulmonary vascular resistance e.g. PE, hypoxia
- Chronic pulmonary venous hypertension e.g. LVF, lung disease.

Causes of pulmonary hypertension
- *Idiopathic*
- *Lung disease:* Asthma, COPD, bronchiectasis, pulmonary fibrosis
- *Cardiac disease:* Mitral stenosis, congenital heart disease, severe LVF
- *Hypoventilation:* Sleep apnoea, enlarged adenoids in children, CVA
- *Pulmonary vascular disease:* PE, sickle-cell disease
- *Neuromuscular disease:* MND, polio, myaesthenia gravis
- *Thoracic cage abnormalities:* Kyphosis, scoliosis
- *Drug induced:* anorectic agents, amphetamines.

Consequences of pulmonary hypertension
- With time, ↑ pressure in the pulmonary vascular tree results in permanent damage to smaller pulmonary vessels and pulmonary hypertension becomes irreversible – even if the cause is removed.
- If a shunt is present, when pulmonary > systemic pressure the shunt reverses and the patient becomes cyanotic (Eisenmenger's syndrome).

Diagnosis: Under-diagnosed – delay between onset of symptoms and diagnosis is ~2y.

Presentation: Congestive cardiac failure ± infective bronchitis, chest pain, breathlessness, lethargy and fatigue, haemoptysis, syncope, nausea.

Examination: Check for cyanosis, peripheral oedema, ↑ JVP, 4th heart sound, diastolic murmur from pulmonary regurgitation, hepatomegaly ± ascites, crepitations at lung bases ± pleural effusion.

Investigations
- *CXR:* Cardiomegaly + enlargement of proximal pulmonary arteries
- *ECG:* Right axis deviation, tall peaked P waves and dominant R wave in right precordial leads *or* right bundle branch block

Management: Refer to cardiologist or chest physician. Doppler echo is used to assess ventricular function and pulmonary arterial pressure. In the UK, ongoing care is now organized into designated multidisciplinary pulmonary hypertension units.

Treatment
- Remove the underlying cause if possible (2° pulmonary hypertension)
- Oxygen therapy for symptomatic relief ± diuretics ± anticoagulation
- Vasodilator therapy is useful for primary pulmonary hypertension: prostaglandin analogues, calcium channel blockers, endothelium receptor analogues e.g. bosentan, sildenafil
- Pulmonary thromboendarterectomy may help patients with chronic thromboembolic pulmonary hypertension.

Prognosis: If the cause is irreversible, a steady decline towards cor pulmonale and death is the likely outcome and heart–lung transplantation the only option. However, newer drugs are improving prognosis.

Pulmonary hypertension and pregnancy: Risk of death is high in conditions where pulmonary blood flow cannot be ↑ e.g. Eisenmenger's syndrome (maternal mortality 30–50%); primary pulmonary hypertension (mortality 40–50%).

Management: Specialist obstetric care is required for all patients with a pre-existing cardiac condition. Where possible refer pre-conception to a cardiologist for discussion of risks. Antibiotic prophylaxis is necessary for women with structural cardiac disease for delivery.

Cor pulmonale: Right heart failure as a result of chronic hypoxia causing chronic pulmonary hypertension. Due to diseases of the lung, its vessels or the thoracic cage.

Further information
British Heart Foundation Factfile Pulmonary hypertension (1/2003) 🖥 www.bhf.org.uk
Chapman *et al. Oxford Handbook of Respiratory Medicine* (2005) Oxford University Press ISBN: 0198529775

Pulmonary arterial hypertension
- Idiopathic
- Familial
- Related to: collagen vascular disease, congenital systemic to pulmonary shunts, portal hypertension, HIV, drugs/toxins, possibly amphetamine, cocaine, chemotherapy agents and other heredity disorders

Pulmonary venous hypertension
- Left-sided atrial or ventricular heart disease
- Left-sided valvular heart disease

Pulmonary hypertension associated with hypoxaemia
- COPD
- Interstitial lung disease
- Sleep disordered breathing
- Alveolar hypoventilation disorders
- Chronic high altitude exposure

Pulmonary hypertension due to chronic thrombotic and/or embolic disease

Pulmonary hypertension associated with miscellaneous disorders
- Inflammatory: e.g. sarcoidosis, Langerhans cell histiocytosis
- Extrinsic compression of the central pulmonary veins: fibrosing mediastinitis, lymphadenopathy/tumours

Respiratory tract infections

Respiratory tract infections are very common and can affect any structure from the nose and mouth down to the lungs (Figure 4.9).

The common cold: Acute, usually afebrile, respiratory tract infection.
- *Causes:* Rhino (30–50%), picorna, echo and Coxsackie's viruses. At any one time only a few viruses are prevalent. Similar symptoms are also caused by the adeno and parainfluenza viruses.
- *Spread:* Contaminated secretions on fingers and droplet infection. Most people are infected 2–3x/y.
- *Management:* Advise patients to take plenty of fluids and paracetamol for symptom relief. Usually symptoms resolve in 4–10d.
- *Complications:* Exacerbation of asthma/COPD; 2° infection (bronchitis, pneumonia, conjunctivitis, OM, sinusitis, tonsillitis).

Acute bronchitis: Inflammation of major bronchi. Probably infective cause (viral or bacterial), although pathogens are not always identified. Often follows viral URTI, especially in winter months.

Presentation
- *Symptoms* include cough ± sputum, breathlessness and wheeze.
- *Signs* – may be none. Include wheeze and coarse crepitations.

Management: Acute bronchitis is a self-limiting illness in normally healthy people. Consider:
- Bronchodilators if wheeze is heard
- Antibiotics – may shorten symptoms but weigh benefits against possible side-effects from antibiotics, ↑ in community antibiotic resistance and 'medicalizing' a self-limiting condition. Antibiotics are more likely to be of benefit if the patient has pre-existing cardiac or pulmonary disease, or persistent mucopurulent sputum.
- If recurrent acute bronchitis consider a diagnosis of COPD.

Acute sinusitis: Infection of the paranasal sinuses (maxillary, frontal, ethmoid and/or sphenoid). Usually follows a viral URTI though 10% are due to tooth infection.

Presentation: Frontal headache/facial pain (may be difficult to distinguish from toothache) – typically worse on movement/bending ± purulent nasal discharge ± fever. Often preceded by URTI.

Management: Most sinusitis resolves spontaneously in 7–10d.
- Advise analgesia (paracetamol ± ibuprofen) and fluids for all patients.
- Steam inhalation may help.
- Short courses of decongestants may help but there is very little evidence of effectiveness.
- Steroid nasal sprays (e.g. beclometasone nasal spray 2 puffs to each nostril bd) may help – evidence of effectiveness is limited.

Reserve antibiotics for patients with severe symptoms or symptoms persisting >7d. – there is limited evidence of benefit[C]. If prescribing, use amoxicillin 250–500mg tds or erythromycin 250–500mg qds for 7d. Doxycycline (200mg on day 1 then 100mg od for 6d.) is an alternative.

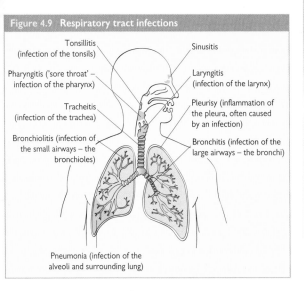

Figure 4.9 Respiratory tract infections

Tonsillitis (infection of the tonsils)

Sinusitis

Pharyngitis ('sore throat' – infection of the pharynx)

Laryngitis (infection of the larynx)

Tracheitis (infection of the trachea)

Pleurisy (inflammation of the pleura, often caused by an infection)

Bronchiolitis (infection of the small airways – the bronchioles)

Bronchitis (infection of the large airways – the bronchi)

Pneumonia (infection of the alveoli and surrounding lung)

GP Notes: Self-help advice to give to patients for management of acute self-limiting upper respiratory tract infections

- Colds and coughs/sinusitis are common and may be caused by viruses or bacteria. Both usually get better without antibiotics.
- You may have other symptoms as well such as fever, tiredness, headache, pain on swallowing and/or swollen glands in your neck.
- Drink plenty of fluids.
- Take paracetamol and/or ibuprofen – taking regular doses works better than just taking doses when you feel you need them.
- Most infections get worse for a few days and then improve and are better within a week or 10 days.
- Contact your GP or NHS Direct if you are worried or want to discuss your symptoms further.

Figure 4.9 is reproduced with permission from 🖥 www.patient.co.uk

Sore throat

Each GP sees ≈120 patients with sore throat every year – mostly children and young adults. 70% sore throats are viral in origin, the rest bacterial (mostly Group A β-haemolytic streptococci).

Clinical picture
- Pain on swallowing
- Fever
- Headache
- Tonsillar exudates
- Nausea and vomiting
- Abdominal pain – especially children due to abdominal lymphadenopathy

Viral and bacterial infections are indistinguishable clinically but association with coryza, and cough, may point to a viral aetiology.

Differential diagnosis: Glandular fever, especially in teenagers with persistent sore throat (send blood for FBC (atypical lymphocytes) and glandular fever antibodies – Monospot or Paul Bunnell – if suspected).

Investigation: Not usually undertaken.
- Throat swabs cannot distinguish commensal organisms (40% carry Group A β-haemolytic streptococci) from clinical infection, are expensive and do not give instant results, so are rarely used.
- Rapid antigen tests give immediate results but have low sensitivity, limiting usefulness.

Management: 90% patients recover within 1 week without treatment. Complications are rare. Advise analgesia and antipyretics (e.g. paracetamol and/or ibuprofen), ↑ fluid intake and salt-water gargles.

Use of antibiotics: Antibiotic prescription can probably be avoided in most patients but educating patients about the reasons for not prescribing is vital to maintain a good doctor–patient relationship.

Benefits of taking antibiotics
- Antibiotics give a modest benefit in symptom relief (8h. less symptoms).
- Antibiotics may confer slight protection against some complications (e.g. quinsy and otitis media). There is no evidence antibiotics protect against rheumatic fever or acute glomerulonephritis.

Risks of taking antibiotics:
- The possibility of side-effects with antibiotic use
- ↑ in community antibiotic resistance
- 'Medicalizing' a self-limiting condition – prescribing ↑ faith in antibiotics and encourages re-attendance with future sore throats

Before prescribing, weigh risks against benefits. If you decide to prescribe antibiotics, use penicillin V or erythromycin 250mg qds for 5–10d. DON'T prescribe amoxicillin as it causes a severe rash if the patient has glandular fever.

An alternative strategy is to issue a 'delayed prescription' for patients to collect if no better in 2–3d. (70% don't collect the script).

Acute epiglottitis: 📖 p.96

GP Notes: Advice for patients (or parents of children) with sore throat

- Sore throat is common and may be caused by viruses or bacteria. Both usually get better without antibiotics.
- You may have other symptoms as well such as cough, fever, tiredness, headache, pain on swallowing and/or swollen glands in your neck.
- Drink plenty of fluids.
- Take paracetamol and/or ibuprofen – taking regular doses works better than just taking doses when you feel you need them.
- Gargles can sometimes sooth the discomfort as well.
- Most sore throats get worse for a few days and then improve and are better within a week.

Figure 4.10 View of the tonsils at examination and acute tonsillitis

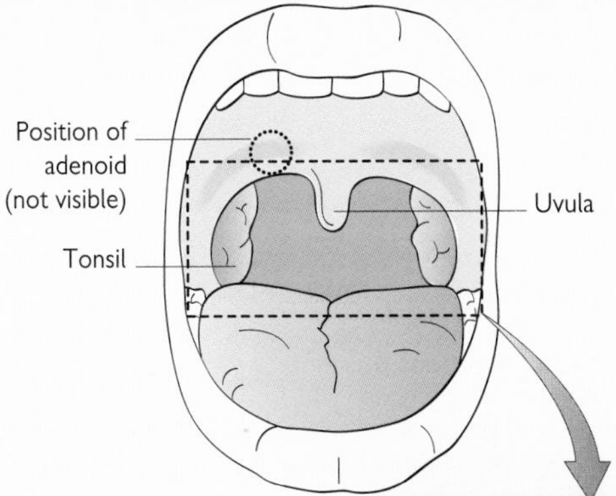
Position of adenoid (not visible)
Uvula
Tonsil

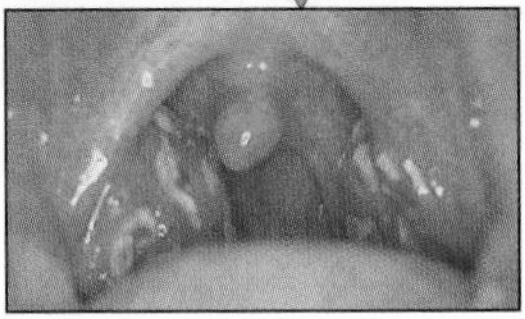

Acute tonsilitis

Complications of sore throat: All rare:
- *Quinsy (peritonsillar abscess):* Usually occurs in adults. *Signs:* Unilateral peritonsillar swelling, difficulty swallowing (even saliva) and trismus (difficulty opening jaw). Refer for IV antibiotics ± incision and drainage.
- *Retropharyngeal abscess:* Occurs in children. *Signs:* inability to swallow, fever. Refer for IV antibiotics ± incision and drainage.
- *Rheumatic fever*
- *Glomerulonephritis*

Indications for referral to ENT

Urgent referral: Any unexplained persistent (>1mo.) sore throat[N].

Referral for tonsillectomy[G]
- *Recurrent acute tonsillitis:* Young children have a lot of throat infections and most will 'grow out' of the problem without the need for surgery. Tonsillectomy is only considered if children miss a lot of school: e.g. >5 attacks causing school absence/y. for 2y.
- *Airway obstruction:* Very large tonsils causing sleep apnoea – 📖 p.97.
- *Chronic tonsillitis:* >3mo. + halitosis.
- *Recurrent quinsy*
- *Unilateral tonsillar enlargement:* To exclude malignancy.

⚠ Tonsillectomy carries a small risk of severe haemorrhage. Readmit any patient with bleeding post-op for observation.

Glandular fever (infectious mononucleosis): Consider in teen-agers or young adults presenting with sore throat lasting >1wk. Caused by Epstein-Barr virus (EBV). Spread by droplet infection and direct contact ('kissing disease') and has a 4–14d. incubation period.

Symptoms/signs: Sore throat, malaise, fatigue, lymphadenopathy, enlarged spleen, palatal petechiae, rash (10–20%).

Investigation: Send blood for FBC (atypical lymphocytes) and glandular fever antibodies (Monospot or Paul-Bunnell).

Management
- Advise rest, fluids and regular paracetamol, avoid alcohol.
- Try salt-water gargles or aspirin gargles (only if >16y.).
- Consider a short course of prednisolone for severe symptoms.
- Treat 2° infection with antibiotics.
- Counsel re the possibility of prolonged symptoms (up to several months).

⚠ DON'T prescribe amoxicillin as it causes a severe rash.

Complications: 2° infections, rash with amoxicillin, hepatitis, jaundice, pneumonitis, neurological disturbances (rare).

Laryngitis: Hoarseness, malaise ± fever and/or pain on using voice. Usually viral and self-limiting (1–2wk.) but occasionally 2° bacterial infection occurs.

Management: Advise patients to rest voice, take OTC analgesia e.g. paracetamol and/or ibuprofen, try steam inhalations. Consider antibiotics if bacterial infection is suspected e.g. penicillin 250mg qds for 1wk.

⚠ Urgent referrals

Refer urgently for chest X-ray (CXR)[N]: ALL patients with hoarseness persisting >3wk. – particularly smokers aged >50y. and heavy drinkers.

If there is a POSITIVE finding on CXR: Refer urgently to a team specializing in the management of lung cancer.

If there is a NEGATIVE finding on CXR: Refer urgently to a team specializing in the management of head and neck cancer.

Refer urgently to ENT[N]: Any unexplained, persistent (>1mo.) sore throat.

Further information

SIGN Management of sore throat and indications for tonsillectomy (1999) 🖳 www.sign.ac.uk

NICE Referral guidelines for suspected cancer – quick reference guide (2005) 🖳 www.nice.org.uk

---

GP Notes: Advice for patients with laryngitis

- Laryngitis is usually caused by a virus and antibiotics do not help.
- It usually settles in about a week.
- Drink plenty of fluids (not tea, coffee, alcohol).
- Rest your voice if possible – avoid shouting, singing or talking for long periods, overuse may make inflammation worse.
- Steam inhalations may help.
- Gargling with aspirin is unlikely to help.
- Take regular paracetamol/ibuprofen for pain, headaches and fever.

Advice for patients: Information for patients

Patient UK Information leaflets on sore throat: UTRI, tonsillitis, laryngitis, tonsils and adenoids, and glandular fever
🖳 www.patient.co.uk

ENT UK Patient information on laryngitis and sore throat
🖳 www.entuk.org

Influenza

Sporadic respiratory illness during autumn and winter causing ≈600 deaths/y. with epidemics every 2–3y. → 10x ↑ in deaths.
- *Causes:* Influenza viruses A, B or C.
- *Spread:* Droplet infection, person-to-person contact, or contact with contaminated items.
- *Incubation:* 1–7d.

Presentation
- In mild cases symptoms are like those of a common cold.
- In more severe cases fever begins suddenly accompanied by prostration and generalized aches and pains.
- Other symptoms may follow: headache, sore throat, respiratory tract symptoms (usually cough ± coryza).
- Acute symptoms resolve in <5d. but weakness, sweating and fatigue may persist longer. 2° chest infection is common.

Management
- ***Symptomatic:*** Rest, fluids and paracetamol for fever/symptom control.
- ***Treatment of secondary complications:*** e.g. antibiotics for chest infection, persistent otitis media or tonsillitis/pharyngitis; treatment of exacerbations of COPD or asthma.
- ***Antivirals:*** Zanamivir (Relenza™ 10mg bd for 5d. by inhalation) and Oseltamivir (Tamiflu™ 75mg bd for 5d.) are not a 'cure' but may shorten duration of symptoms and ↓ incidence of complications if started <48h. after onset of symptoms. Antivirals should only be used for treatment of patients in high-risk groups (Box 4.5 – except pregnancy) and only when influenza is prevalent in the community[N]. Zanamivir should only be used for adults; oseltamivir can be used for adults or children >1y.

148

⚠ Zanamivir may cause bronchospasm – ensure a short-acting bronchodilator is available if the patient has a tendency to bronchospasm. Avoid in severe asthma unless close monitoring and facilities to treat bronchospasm are available.

Prevention
- Influenza vaccine is prepared each year from viruses of the 3 strains thought most likely to cause flu that winter. It is ~70% effective (range 30–90%). Protection lasts 1y. Give to high-risk groups[£] – Box 4.5.
- Oseltamivir is recommended for prophylaxis in high-risk patients >13y. who are not effectively vaccinated or who live in residential care where a staff member has influenza-like symptoms only when influenza is prevalent in the community. Use at a dose of 75mg od for 7–10d. from diagnosis of the latest case in the establishment[N].

ⓘ Community-based virological surveillance schemes will indicate when influenza is circulating in the community.

GMS contract

Influenza vaccination

CHD 12	% of patients with CHD who have a record of influenza immunization in the preceding 1 September–31 March	up to 7 points	40–90%
Stroke 10	% of patients with TIA/stroke who have a record of influenza immunization in the preceding 1 September–31 March	up to 2 points	40–85%
Diabetes 18	% of patients with diabetes who have a record of influenza immunization in the preceding 1 September–31 March	up to 3 points	40–85%
COPD 8	% of COPD patients who have a record of influenza immunization in the preceding 1 September–31 March	up to 6 points	40–85%

Influenza vaccination may be offered by GMS practices as a directed enhanced service – 📖 p.246

Box 4.5

Patients at risk of developing severe disease with influenza

- Aged ≥65y. or
- With ≥1 of the following conditions:
  - Chronic respiratory disease including COPD and asthma
  - Significant cardiovascular disease excluding hypertension
  - Chronic renal disease
  - Immunosuppression (including hyposplenism)
  - Diabetes mellitus.

Indications for influenza vaccination

- ≥65y.
- Chronic renal disease
- DM
- Chronic liver disease
- Chronic lung disease e.g. asthma, COPD
- Cardiovascular disease (except ↑BP alone)
- Immunocompromised or asplenic patients
- Carers of patients with disabilities
- Patients living in long-stay residential care establishments
- Health professionals expected to be in contact with influenza

149

Further information

NICE Guidance on the use of zanamivir, oseltamivir and amantadine for the treatment of influenza (2003) 🖥 www.nice.org.uk
Health Protection Agency (HPA) Topics A–Z: Influenza 🖥 www.hpa.org.uk

Influenza pneumonia: The principal viral cause of pneumonia is influenza A virus. This usually occurs during epidemics of influenza A – Asian flu – but is rare. May affect previously healthy individuals but patients with underlying disease e.g. COPD are at greater risk. Features:
- Develops rapidly
- Presents with progressive dyspnoea
- Acute haemorrhagic disease of the lungs may cause death within hours
- Treatment is supportive and, if detected early enough, with antivirals.

🛈 The most common cause of pneumonia during influenza epidemics is secondary bacterial infection, usually with *Staphylococcus aureus* or *Streptococcus pneumoniae*.

Bird flu
- A severe form of avian influenza or 'bird flu' – called H5N1 – has affected poultry flocks and other birds since 2003.
- As of December 2005, 138 people have also caught the infection, as a result of close and direct contact with infected birds. 71 have subsequently died.
- There is no firm evidence that H5N1 has acquired the ability to pass easily from person to person.
- Concern remains that the virus might develop the ability to pass from person to person, or that it might mix with human flu viruses to create a new virus and create a new human flu pandemic.

150

GP Notes: Recommendations for travellers to areas experiencing outbreaks of bird flu in poultry

- Avoid visiting live animal markets and poultry farms.
- Avoid contact with surfaces contaminated with animal faeces.
- Do not attempt to bring any live poultry products back to the UK.

Further information
DOH (Chief Medical Officer) Explaining pandemic flu (2005). Available from 🖳 www.dh.gov.uk

Advice for patients: Advice about bird flu

You can reduce, but not eliminate, the risk of catching or spreading influenza during a pandemic by

- covering your nose and mouth when coughing or sneezing, and using a tissue when possible
- disposing of dirty tissues promptly and carefully – bag and bin them
- avoiding non-essential travel and large crowds whenever possible
- maintaining good basic hygiene, for example washing your hands frequently with soap and water to reduce the spread of the virus from your hands to your face, or to other people
- cleaning hard surfaces (e.g. kitchen worktops, door handles) frequently, using a normal cleaning product
- making sure your children follow this advice.

If you do catch flu

- stay at home and rest
- take medicines such as aspirin, ibuprofen or paracetamol to relieve the symptoms – follow the instructions with the medicines
- drink plenty of fluids.

❶ Children under 16 must not be given aspirin or ready-made flu remedies containing aspirin.

These measures are for your own health and to avoid spreading the illness to others.

Should a flu pandemic occur, more information will be given through leaflets, websites and the media. It will tell you more about how you can protect yourself and your family and what to do if you think you are infected. Special treatment will be recommended for some people at greatest risk from flu and further information about treatment will be given at that time.

151

Advice is reproduced with permission from *Bird Flu and Pandemic Influenza: what are the risks?* (DoH, 2005) 🖥 www.dh.gov.uk

Pneumonia

Common condition with annual incidence of ~8 cases/1000 adult population. Incidence ↑ with age and peaks in the winter. Mortality for those managed in the community is <1% but 1 in 4 patients with pneumonia are admitted to hospital and mortality for those admitted is ~9%.

Presentation: Acute illness characterized by:
- Symptoms of an acute lower respiratory tract illness (cough + ≥1 other lower respiratory tract symptom e.g. purulent sputum, pleurisy)
- New focal chest signs on examination (consolidation or ↓ air entry, coarse crackles and/or pleural rub)
- ≥1 systemic feature:
  - Sweating, fevers, shivers, aches and pains *and/or*
  - Temperature ≥38°C
- No other explanation for the illness.

ⓘ The elderly may present atypically e.g. 'off legs' or acute confusion.

Investigations: Often unnecessary in general practice. Consider:
- *Pulse oximetry* (if available): Use to assess severity. If oxygen saturation ≤92% in air, the patient is hypoxic and requires admission
- *CXR:* If diagnostic uncertainty or symptoms not resolving. CXR changes may lag behind clinical signs but should return to normal <6wk. after recovery. Persistent changes on CXR >6wk. after recovery require further investigation
- *Sputum culture:* If not responding to treatment. If weight ↓, malaise, night sweats or risk factors for TB (ethnic origin, history of TB exposure, social deprivation or elderly), request mycobacterium culture
- *Blood:* FBC: ↑ WCC; ESR ↑; acute and convalescent titres to confirm 'atypical' pneumonia (*Legionella, C. Psittaci, M. pneumonia*).

Differential diagnosis
- Pneumonitis e.g. 2° to radiotherapy, chemical inhalation
- Pulmonary oedema (may coexist in the elderly)
- PE
- Acute bronchitis
- Exacerbation of COPD
- Lung cancer
- Bronchiectasis

TB: 📖 p.158

Further information
British Thoracic Society Guidelines for the management of community-acquired pneumonia in adults (2001) and Update (2004) 🖥 www.brit-thoracic.org.uk
Chapman *et al. Oxford Handbook of Respiratory Medicine* (2005) Oxford University Press ISBN: 0198529775

Table 4.9 Common causative organisms

Organism (%)	Features
Streptococcus pneumoniae (36%)	Most common cause of lobar pneumonia. Vaccination is protective. More common in patients with DM and alcoholics. Usually penicillin-sensitive in the community. Treat with amoxicillin 250–500mg tds or erythromycin 250–500mg qds.
Haemophilus influenzae (10%)	More common amongst the elderly, patients in nursing homes and patients with COPD. Organisms are often penicillin-resistant (15%). Treat with erythromycin 250–500mg qds for 1wk.
Influenza A&B (8%)	Annual epidemics in the winter months. ~3% develop pneumonia. Risk factors include: • Chronic respiratory disease including COPD and asthma • Significant cardiovascular disease excluding hypertension • Chronic renal disease • Immunosuppression (including hyposplenism) • Diabetes mellitus.
Mycoplasma pneumoniae (1.3%)	Less common in the elderly. Epidemics occur ~ every 4y. in the UK. Treat with erythromycin 250–500mg qds for 2wk.
Gram-negative enteric bacteria (1.3%)	Associated with aspiration. Organisms are usually sensitive to co-amoxiclav 250/125 tds or penicillin V 250–500mg qds + metronidazole 400mg tds.
Chlamydia species (1.3%)	~20% have history of bird contact (associated with C. psittaci infection). Treat with erythromycin 250–500mg qds for 2wk. or azithromycin 500mg od for 3d. Tetracycline is an alternative.
Staphylococcus aureus (0.8%)	More common in the winter months. May be associated with viral infection e.g. flu, measles. Treat with penicillin V 250–500mg and flucloxacillin 250–500mg qds for 2–3wk.
Legionella species (0.4%)	Most common in September/October. >50% are related to travel. More common amongst patients on oral steroids or immunosuppressed. Treatment is with erythromycin 250–500mg qds for 3wk. Rifampicin may be needed in addition for severe infections.
Moraxella catarrhalis	Causes bronchitis or pneumonia in children and adults with underlying chronic lung disease.
Pseudomonas aeruginosa	Causes pneumonia in patients with immunosuppression and chronic lung disease (particularly CF – may cause chronic infection). Always needs specialist management.

Management:

Consider the need for admission: Figure 4.11
- Have a low threshold for admission if:
  - Ill but apyrexial
  - Concomitant illness (e.g. CCF, chronic lung, renal or liver disease, DM, cancer) *or*
  - Poor social situation.
- If life-threatening infection or considerable delay (>2h.) consider administering antibiotics before admission.

If a decision is made to treat at home:
- Advise not to smoke, to rest and drink plenty of fluids.
- Start antibiotics e.g. amoxicillin 500mg–1g tds, erythromycin 500mg tds or clarithromycin 500mg bd.
- Treat pleuritic pain with simple analgesia e.g. paracetamol 1g qds.
- Review within 48h. Reassess clinical state.
- If deteriorating or not improving consider CXR or admission.

Possible reasons why patients may not improve:
- Elderly – slow clinical response
- Incorrect diagnosis (see differential diagnosis – 📖 p.152)
- Incorrect antibiotics e.g. antibiotic resistance
- Non-bacterial cause e.g. viral, fungal
- TB
- Impaired immunity e.g. HIV
- Secondary complication

Complications: Require specialist management – refer.
- *Pleural effusion:* May be reactive or empyema (pus in the lung cavity)
- *Lung abscess:* May be single/multiple. Presents with swinging fever and worsening cough/breathlessness ± haemoptyisis ± foul sputum. Often the result of aspiration pneumonia and shares the same risk factors (📖 p.156)
- *Respiratory failure:* Adult respiratory distress syndrome
- *Septicaemia*
- *Metastatic infection:* e.g. meningitis, endocarditis, septic arthritis
- *Renal failure*
- *MI*
- *Jaundice*

Prevention: Vaccination of high-risk individuals:

Influenza vaccination: 📖 p.149

Pneumococcal vaccination: Routine vaccination will be offered as part of the childhood immunization schedule in the near future. Meanwhile, offer to high-risk patients (Box 4.6). Children receive pneumococcal vaccination as part of the routine vaccination programme at 2, 4 and 12 Mo. A catch-up programme will immunize all children <2y. who have not been vaccinated. Ineffective aged <2mo.
🛈 Booster doses are not needed except for patients with asplenia or nephrotic syndrome – when give a booster after 5–10y.

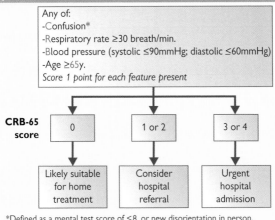

Figure 4.11 Assessment of severity and management of pneumonia

Any of:
-Confusion*
-Respiratory rate ≥30 breath/min.
-Blood pressure (systolic ≤90mmHg; diastolic ≤60mmHg)
-Age ≥65y.
Score 1 point for each feature present

CRB-65 score

| 0 | 1 or 2 | 3 or 4 |

| Likely suitable for home treatment | Consider hospital referral | Urgent hospital admission |

*Defined as a mental test score of ≤8, or new disorientation in person, place or time.

Box 4.6 High-risk patients for pneumococcal infection

- ≥65y. of age
- Asplenia or functional asplenia (📖 p.165) e.g. splenectomy, sickle cell
- Chronic renal disease or nephrotic syndrome
- Immunodeficiency or immunosuppression e.g. lymphoma, Hodgkin's disease, multiple myeloma, HIV, chemotherapy
- Chronic heart disease, lung disease (e.g. asthma, COPD) or liver disease
- Coeliac disease
- Cochlear implant
- DM
- CSF shunts
- Children <5y. who have had previous invasive pneumococcal disease

Further information
British Thoracic Society: Guidelines for the management of community-acquired pneumonia in adults (2001) and Update (2004) 🖥 www.brit-thoracic.org.uk

GMS contract

Influenza and pneumococcal vaccination may be offered by GMS practices as a directed enhanced service – 📖 p.246

Figure 4.11 is reproduced with permission from the British Thoracic Society

Aspiration pneumonia: Lung infection resulting from aspiration of organisms into the lower respiratory tract – right lung > left lung. Risk of infection is related to volume of fluid aspirated. Infection is usually with anaerobes ± Gram –ve enteric bacteria.

Patients at risk of aspiration pneumonia: Include:
- Patients with a reduced conscious level e.g. due to alcohol, as a result of drugs (including anaesthesia), associated with seizures, during sleep
- Depressed gag reflex – stroke, bulbar palsy (e.g. due to MND)
- Gastro-oesophageal reflux or vomiting
- Upper GI abnormalities e.g. oesophageal stricture, tracheo-oesophageal fistula
- NG tube feeding.

Presentation:
- Cough, fever, dyspnoea and purulent sputum.
- In the elderly may present insidiously with low-grade fever, malaise, weight loss and anaemia/↑ WCC.
- Untreated, the condition may progress to lung abscess/bronchiectasis.

Management: Treatment: is with co-amoxiclav 250/125 tds or metronidazole 400mg tds + penicillin 250–500mg qds

ⓘ If the cause of aspiration is not clear, refer for speech therapy review to assess swallowing and/or neurological review.

Viral pneumonia: Rare in comparison with bacterial pneumonia or viral URTI. Usually presents with worsening cough, breathlessness ± wheeze. Diagnosis is confirmed by a rise in specific antibody titre.
- Influenza is the most common cause of viral pneumonia in adults in the UK (📖 p.150).
- Adeno virus may cause pneumonia in young adults.
- Pneumonia complicates chickenpox in 5–14% adult chickenpox infections. Chest symptoms develop several days after the rash appears. Pneumonia is likely to be more severe with ↑ mortality in patients who are pregnant, immunocompromised due to disease or treatment, or on steroid treatment. Refer for same-day CXR or admit if suspected. Treatment is with IV aciclovir.
- Measles virus may cause pneumonia at any age, though 2° bacterial pneumonia is more common.
- Respiratory syncitial virus (RSV) and cytomegalovirus (CMV) cause pneumonia in patients who are immunocompromised due to drugs or disease.

Pneumocystis carinii (PCP): 📖 p.162

Sudden acute respiratory syndrome (SARS): 📖 p.162

GP Notes: Chickenpox pneumonia

Chickenpox in pregnancy: Contact with chickenpox in pregnancy is common. If the mother has definitely had chickenpox there is no risk to herself or the baby. If she doesn't recall having chickenpox, check her immunity with a blood test – 80% have antibodies from silent infection.

Risk to the mother: Chickenpox pneumonia is more common and can be severe.

Risks to the baby
- *<20wk. gestation* – 1–2% risk of chickenpox syndrome: eye defects, hypoplasia, microcephaly. If a woman has varicella-zoster Ig (VZ-Ig) treatment (see below) after being exposed, risk is even lower.
- *Mother's rash develops <1wk. prior to delivery to 1mo. after delivery* – risk of overwhelming infection. Baby may need VZ-Ig treatment.

Management
- In cases of 'at risk' exposure, arrange for VZ-Ig to be given to mother and/or baby. This can be life-saving and significantly ↓ disease severity. It must be given ≤10d. after exposure.
- If the mother develops chickenpox take expert advice. Treatment is usually with aciclovir if the mother presents <24h. after rash appears and is >20wk. gestation.

Chickenpox in immunocompromised patients
- In cases of 'at risk' exposure, arrange for VZ-Ig to be given. This can be life-saving and significantly ↓ disease severity. It must be given ≤10d. after exposure.
- If the patient develops chickenpox take expert advice. Treatment is usually with IV aciclovir.

Further information
RCOG Chickenpox in pregnancy (2001) 🖥 www.rcog.org.uk
DTB Chickenpox, pregnancy and the newborn (2005) **45**(9): 69–72.

Tuberculosis[ND]

Caused by *Mycobacterium tuberculosis*. Worldwide 1½ billion people have tuberculosis (TB). In the UK 7000 cases of TB are reported each year and 350 patients die. Incidence is increasing and 10% cases are antibiotic resistant.

Risk factors: In the UK:
- 40% cases of TB occur in London. TB is an urban disease
- 70% cases occur in ethnic minority populations – 60% in those born abroad ($^1/_2$ are diagnosed <5y. after entering the country)
- Contacts of other patients with TB:
  - If living in the same house risk is 1:3
  - If school/work contact risk is up to 1:50
  - Casual social contact risk is 1:100,000
- Immunnosuppressed patients – especially patients with HIV
- Homeless people.

Primary TB: Initial infection. Transmitted by droplet infection. A lesion forms (usually pulmonary) which drains to local LNs. Immunity develops and the infection becomes quiescent.

Symptoms/signs: May be none. Fever, night sweats, persistent cough ± sputum/haemoptysis, pneumonia and/or pleural effusion, anorexia and weight loss, erythema nodosum.

Investigations: CXR, sputum samples for culture (state on the form that you are looking for acid-fast bacilli), tuberculin test +ve (may be –ve if immunocompromised) lymphadenopathy.

Management: Refer for treatment and contact tracing.

Post-primary TB: Reactivation of a primary infection. Initial lesions – usually in the upper lobes of the lung – progress and fibrose. Other sites may develop disease. Multiple small lesions throughout the body result in miliary TB and are common in immunocompromised patients. Symptoms and signs relate to the organs infected.

Extrapulmonary disease sites:
- CNS
- Lymph nodes
- Pericardium
- Spine (rarely other bones/joints)
- Peripheral cold abscess
- Miliary

Risk factors
- Old age
- Malignancy
- DM
- Steroids
- HIV
- Poor nutrition
- Chronic illness

Management: Refer for specialist treatment.

Screening: TB is a notifiable disease. Every time a case of TB is notified, contact tracing is initiated – usually through chest clinics. All contacts are screened for TB with a tuberculin test (Table 4.10). Screen other high-risk groups before vaccination.

GP Notes: Tuberculin skin test

Useful in diagnosis of TB and must be carried out before BCG immunization, except for infants <3mo. old who have not had any recent contact with TB. The Mantoux test (international standard) is replacing the Heaf test as the standard method of tuberculin skin testing in the UK in 2005/2006.

Interpretation: Table 4.10

False results: The tuberculin test can be suppressed by:
- Glandular fever infection
- Viral infections
- Live viral vaccines – don't do a tuberculin test <3wk. after vaccination
- Hodgkin's disease
- Sarcoidosis
- Corticosteroid therapy
- Immunosuppressant treatment or diseases, including HIV.

⚠ If a patient has a +ve tuberculin test, DON'T give BCG vaccination.

Table 4.10 Tuberculin testing and interpretation of results

Heaf test	Mantoux test	Grade
No induration at puncture sites	0mm induration	0 – Negative
Discrete induration at ≥4 sites	1–4mm induration	1 – Negative
Ring of induration with clear centre	5–14mm induration	2 – Positive*
Disc of induration 5–10mm wide	≥15mm induration	3 – Refer to chest clinic
Solid induration>10mm wide ± vesiculation or ulceration		4 – Refer to chest clinic

* In schoolchildren, a grade 2 response requires no further action. In other circumstances, refer to a chest clinic.

159

Treatment[G]: ⚠ Always refer to the chest clinic

Asymptomatic people with +ve tuberculin skin test (Mantoux >10mm) but normal CXR: are treated with isoniazid for 6mo. or isoniazid + rifampicin for 3mo. to prevent development of the clinical disease.

Treatment of symptomatic patients: Combination of 3–4 antibiotics for the 1st 2mo. then 2 antibiotics for a further 4mo. Antibiotics used are rifampicin, isoniazid, pyrazinamide and ethambutol. All have potentially serious side-effects and require blood monitoring. Compliance is imperative to prevent antibiotic resistance. Those found to be non-compliant are best treated with Directly Observed Therapy (DOT), in which drugs are dispensed by and taken in the presence of a health professional.

Prevention
- BCG vaccination is vaccination with a live attenuated strain of bacteria derived from *M. bovis*.
- BCG vaccination provides immunity lasting ≥15y. to 70–80% of recipients.
- It is given by intradermal injection into the left upper arm.

⚠ Don't give other immunizations into the same arm for 3mo. after BCG vaccination.

Target groups: The routine screening and vaccination of all school-children is changing to targeted immunization of:
- All infants living in areas where incidence of TB is ≥40/100,000
- Infants whose parents or grandparents were born in a country with TB incidence of ≥40/100,000
- Previously unvaccinated new immigrants from countries where there is a high prevalence of TB
- Those at risk due to their occupation e.g. health care workers, veterinary staff, prison staff.
- Contacts of known cases
- Those living or working in high-prevalence countries for extended periods (generally ≥1mo.).

Children who would otherwise have been offered screening and vaccination as part of the school vaccination programme will be screened for risk factors and tested and vaccinated as needed.

Further information
NICE Tuberculosis (2006) 🖥 www.nice.org.uk
British Thoracic Society 🖥 www.brit-thoracic.org.uk
- Chemotherapy and management of tuberculosis in the UK *Thorax* (1998) **53**(7): 536–48.
- Control and prevention of tuberculosis in the UK: code of practice. *Thorax* (2000) **55**: 887–901.

Health Protection Agency (HPA) Topics A–Z: Tuberculosis.
🖥 www.hpa.org.uk
DoH *Stopping Tuberculosis in England: an action plan from the Chief Medical Officer* (2004) 🖥 www.dh.gov.uk

Advice for patients: Information for patients

Immunization NHS website for patients
🖥 www.immunisation.org.uk
Health Protection Agency (HPA) TB and BCG 🖥 www.hpa.org.uk
British Lung Foundation ☎ 08458 50 50 20 🖥 www.lunguk.org

Other infections

Aspergillosis: A spectrum of diseases. *Cause: Aspergillus* fungus present in the soil and decaying vegetation. Its spores can be inhaled any time of the year but reach peak levels in autumn and winter. Inhaled fungal spores colonize bronchial mucosa and nasal sinuses. If suspected refer to a chest physician.

Presentations
- *Extrinsic asthma:* 📖 p.104
- *Allergic bronchopulmonary aspergillosis:* Grows in the walls of the bronchi. Presents with episodes of eosinophilic pneumonia (characterized by wheeze, cough, fever and malaise) throughout the year but worse in late autumn. CXR shows fleeting lung shadows (cleared by expectorating firm, brown plugs of mucus). Untreated → upper lobe fibrosis and 'proximal' bronchiectasis.
- *Invasive aspergillosis:* Only occurs in the immunocompromised. Aspergillus disseminates from the lung → brain, kidneys and other organs. Carries very poor prognosis.
- *Aspergillus sinusitis:* Nasal congestion, headache and facial discomfort.
- *Aspergilloma:* Growth within existing lung cavities (e.g. from previous TB or sarcoidosis). A ball of fungus forms. CXR shows a round lesion with air halo above it. Occasionally results in haemoptysis.

Management: Refer for specialist management.

Pneumocystis jiroveci (formerly known as PCP): May be classified as a protozoan or fungus. Causes pneumonia in immunocompromised patients.
- *Presentation:* Fever, breathlessness, tachypnoea, dry cough, respiratory failure (± cyanosis).
- *Investigation:* CXR normal or 'ground glass' appearance; sputum culture may be diagnostic.
- *Management:* If suspected refer for specialist care. Treatment is with septrin or dapsone.
- *Prevention:* Prophylactic antibiotics (usually co-trimoxazole) are given to AIDS patients with CD4 counts <200cells/mm^3.

Sudden acute respiratory syndrome (SARS): SARS was first reported in China in 2002. Since then there have been several further clusters in Far East Asia and one in Canada. SARS is caused by a corona virus (SARS-CoV) and spread by direct contact with an infected individual or rarely aerosol transmission. Incubation is 2–10d.

2 stages
- Prodrome – fever (>38°C), malaise, headache, myalgia.
- Respiratory phase – develops after 3–7d. – dry cough and breathlessness. A high proportion progress to respiratory failure. 70% also develop diffuse watery diarrhoea.

🛈 Cases in the UK are most likely to occur within 10d. of return from an affected area, especially one where transmission is thought to be continuing. Admit to a specialist infectious diseases unit. Symptomatic suspected cases should wear a surgical mask during transit.

Further information

Health Protection Agency (HPA) Topics A–Z: Aspergillus; Pneumocystis carinii; SARS 🖥 www.hpa.org.uk

The Aspergillus Website 🖥 www.aspergillus.man.ac.uk

Infections in immunocompromised patients

Infections in patients whose host defence mechanisms are compromised range from minor to fatal. They are often are caused by organisms that normally reside on body surfaces.

Opportunistic infections: Infections from endogenous microflora that are nonpathogenic or from ordinarily harmless organisms. Occur if host defence mechanisms have been altered by:

- Age
- Infection
- Burns
- Neoplasms
- Metabolic disorders
- Irradiation
- Foreign bodies
- Corticosteroids
- Immunosuppressive or cytotoxic drugs
- Diagnostic or therapeutic instrumentation

The precise character of the host's altered defences determines which organisms are likely to be involved. These organisms are often resistant to multiple antibiotics.

Organisms commonly involved

- Non-pathogenic streptococci
- E. coli
- Herpes viruses
- Cytomegalovirus
- Cryptococcal infection
- Toxoplasma
- Mycobacteria – 📖 p.158
- Pneumocystis – 📖 p.162
- Candida

Management: Expert care is always required – refer promptly to the consultant responsible for the patient.

Prophylaxis

Antibiotics: Used for prevention of:
- Rheumatic fever and bacterial endocarditis
- TB and meningitis in exposed patients
- Recurrent UTIs and otitis media
- Bacterial infections in granulocytopenic patients
- Pneumocystis (if CD4 count <200cells/mm^3), toxoplasma (if CD4 count <100cells/mm^3) and mycobacterium avium (if CD4 count <50cells/mm^3) in AIDS patients.

⚠ Watch for signs of superinfection with resistant organisms.

Active immunization:
- *Influenza vaccine:* Give annually – see 📖 p.148 for list of indications.
- *Haemophilus influenzae type b vaccine:* For asplenic/hyposplenic patients – children should complete routine Hib vaccinations. Individuals immunized in infancy who then become asplenic should receive 1 booster dose aged >1y. Unimmunized adults and children >10y. should receive a single dose of Hib.
- *Meningococcal vaccine:* Give to close contacts of patients with type A or C meningococcal meningitis. In some cases given to patients with immunosuppression – take specialist advice.

- *Pneumococcal vaccine:* Single dose – give to chronically ill, asplenic and elderly patients and those with sickle-cell and HIV disease. Booster doses are not required except for patients with asplenia or nephrotic syndrome when a booster should be given after 5–10y.
- *Hepatitis B vaccine:* Give to patients who repeatedly receive blood products as well as to medical and nursing personnel and others at risk.

Passive immunization: Can prevent or ameliorate herpes zoster (VZ-Ig), hepatitis A and B, measles and cytomegalovirus infection in selected immunosuppressed patients. If a patient is in contact with any of these diseases, ask advice from the consultant looking after the patient or a consultant in communicable disease control.

Immunoglobulin administration: Effective for patients with hypogammaglobulinaemia. Given on a regular basis by IV infusion.

⚠

- Warn patients about risk of severe malaria and other tropical infections.
- Admit patients to hospital if infection develops despite prophylactic measures.

Asplenic patients: All asplenic patients (or functionally asplenic patients e.g. patients with sickle-cell disease) are at ↑ risk of bacterial infection. Ensure patients have:

- *Vaccinations:* Haemophilus influenzae b, pneumococcal, influenza and, in some cases, meningococcal vaccine. If possible, vaccinations should be given >2wk. prior to splenectomy.
- *Prophylactic antibiotics:* Oral penicillin continuously until age 16y. or for 2y. post-splenectomy – whichever is longer.
- *Stand-by amoxicillin:* To start if symptoms of infection begin.
- *Patient-held card:* Alerting health professionals to infection risk.

GP Notes:

Patient cards and information sheets about hyposplenism/asplenism are available from: Department of Health, PO Box 410, Wetherby LS23 7LL.

Encourage patients to wear a Medic-Alert bracelet or necklace.

GMS contract

Vaccinations can be provided as

- *An additional service* (📖 p.246) – opting out of giving vaccinations to the under 5's results in a 1% ↓ in global sum and opting out of giving other essential vaccinations results in a 2% ↓ in global sum.
- *A directed enhanced service* (📖 p.246) – a payment is available for reaching vaccination targets for Hib vaccination for children aged 2, and offering influenza and pneumococcal vaccination.

165

Bronchiectasis

Bronchiectasis is irreversible dilation of bronchi due to inflammatory destruction of the bronchial wall. This results in impaired clearance of secretions which predisposes to further infection and more damage.

Causes: An underlying cause is found in only 50% of cases:
- *Congenital* – CF, Kartagener syndrome, primary ciliary dyskinesia, Young syndrome
- *Post-infection* – TB, pertussis, measles, pneumonia, bronchopulmonary aspergillosis
- *Immune dysfunction* – HIV, chronic lymphocytic leukaemia, hypogammaglobulinaemia
- *Bronchial obstruction* – foreign body, tumour, extrinsic compression (e.g. from lymph nodes)
- *Toxicity* – inhalation, aspiration
- *Other* – associated with some systemic diseases e.g. rheumatoid arthritis (35% have bronchiectasis), connective tissue diseases, inflammatory bowel disease, Marfan's syndrome, yellow nail syndrome.

Presentation: Consider in any patient with persistent or recurrent chest infections.
- *Mild cases* – asymptomatic with winter exacerbations consisting of fever, cough, purulent sputum, pleuritic chest pain, dyspnoea
- *More severe cases* – persistent cough and sputum, haemoptysis, clubbing, low-pitched inspiratory and expiratory crackles and wheeze.

Investigations
- CXR (abnormalities in 50% cases)
- Sputum – M,C&S – include atypical organisms, acid-fast bacilli and *Aspergillus*
- Spirometry – reversible airways obstruction is common
- CT scan – high-resolution CT scanning detects disease in 97% cases

Management: Refer to a respiratory physician. Treatment aims to improve symptoms, ↓ exacerbations and ↓ progression/mortality. Options include:
- Treatment of the underlying condition (if possible)
- Physiotherapy
- Antibiotics
- Bronchodilators
- Vaccination – advise influenza and pneumococcal vaccination
- Surgery (rarely) – transplant.

Complications
- Chronic infection
- Recurrent pneumonia
- Haemoptysis – can be massive
- Pneumothorax
- Lung abscess
- Respiratory failure

Kartagener syndrome (immotile cilia syndrome): Combination of bronchiectasis, chronic sinusitis and male infertility plus situs inversus (transposed heart and abdominal organs). Due to defect in cilia function. Otitis media and salpingitis are frequent.

Young's syndrome: Bronchiectasis, sinusitis and obstructive azoo-spermia. Often first diagnosed in middle-aged men.

Primary ciliary dyskinesia: Rare autosomal recessive condition. 30% have situs inversus. Other features include:
- Rhinitis
- Persistent wet cough
- Glue ear in childhood
- Wheeze (20%)
- ♂ infertility

Pleural effusion

Fluid in the pleural cavity (Figure 4.12). Simple effusions may be transudates (<30g/l protein) or exudates (>30g/l protein). Alternatively effusions can be made of blood, lymph or pus (empyema).

Causes of simple effusion
- Malignancy (lung cancer, mesothelioma, Meig's syndrome, lymphangitis, lymphoma, metastatic cancer)
- Infection (e.g. pneumonia, TB)
- Heart failure
- Inflammation (SLE, RA, pancreatitis, asbestos exposure)
- Infarction (PE)
- Constrictive pericarditis
- Hypoproteinaemia (e.g. nephrotic syndrome liver disease)
- Hypothyroidism
- Sub-diaphragmatic causes (e.g. intra-abdominal infection)

Presentation
Symptoms: May be an incidental finding on CXR. Symptoms include:
- Dyspnoea
- Pleuritic pain
- Symptoms of underlying cause.

Signs:
- Absent breath sounds
- Dullness to percussion
- ↓ tactile vocal fremitus
- ↓ vocal resonance
- Above the effusion there is usually a zone of bronchial breathing
- Early on there may be a pleural rub
- Large effusions shift the mediastinum away from the affected side and there may be ↓ chest wall movement

Investigations: Confirmed on CXR. If cause is not immediately apparent refer for diagnostic tap (should be done where X-ray facilities are available).

Management: Treat the underlying cause. Refer for drainage if symptomatic. Repeated drainage ± pleurodesis may be necessary.

Further information
British Thoracic Society Guidelines for the management of pleural effusion (2003) ⊞ www.brit-thoracic.org.uk

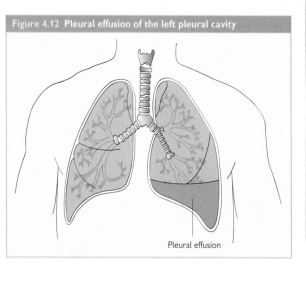

Figure 4.12 Pleural effusion of the left pleural cavity

Pleural effusion

Lung cancer

Commonest cancer (37,000 cases/y.) and 3rd most common cause of death in the UK. Incidence ↑ with age – 85% are aged >65y. and 1% <40y. at presentation. ♂:♀ ≈ 2:1 but incidence is increasing in women.

Types
- *Small-cell lung cancer:* Accounts for ~¼ all cases. Often disseminated by the time of diagnosis. Spreads to liver, bones, brain and adrenals.
- *Non-small-cell lung cancer:* Mainly adenocarcinoma or squamous cell carcinoma. Not always smoking related.

Screening: A 2003 Cochrane review concluded that current evidence does not support screening for lung cancer with chest radiography or sputum cytology. Frequent chest X-ray screening might be harmful. Results of trials of screening with CT scanning are awaited from the US but preliminary results do not suggest this will be an effective screening strategy.

Prevention
- *Smoking cessation* (📖 pp.137–8): 90% of lung cancer patients are smokers or ex-smokers.
- *Diet*: ↑ consumption of fruit, carrots & green vegetables may ↓ incidence but there is no evidence that vitamin supplements are beneficial and they might be harmful[C].

Presentation: >90% have symptoms at the time of diagnosis. Common presenting features:
- Cough (56%)
- Chest/shoulder pain (37%)
- Haemoptysis (7%)
- Dyspnoea
- Hoarseness
- Weight ↓
- Finger clubbing
- General malaise
- Distant metastases
- Incidental finding on CXR

Management: Once the diagnosis has been confirmed, liaise with the chest physician, specialist lung cancer team, primary health care team and specialist palliative care services (e.g. Macmillan nurses). Active treatment options depend on type and extent of tumour and include surgery, radiotherapy and/or chemotherapy. Follow up regularly. 80% die in <1y.

Palliative care: 📖 p.190

Pancoast syndrome: Apical lung cancer + ipsilateral Horner's syndrome. *Cause:* invasion of the cervical sympathetic plexus. *Other features:* shoulder and arm pain (brachial plexus invasion C8-T2) ± hoarse voice/bovine cough (unilateral recurrent laryngeal nerve palsy and vocal cord paralysis).

Further information
NICE Referral guidelines for suspected cancer – quick reference guide (2005) 🖥 www.nice.org.uk
SIGN Management of lung cancer (1998) 🖥 www.sign.ac.uk

GMS contract

Cancer 1	The practice can produce a register of all cancer patients (excluding non-melanotic skin cancer) diagnosed after 1.4.2003	5 points	
Cancer 3	% of patients with cancer diagnosed within 18mo. who have a patient review recorded as occuring <6mo. after the practice received confirmation of diagnosis	up to 6 points	40–90%
Education 7	The practice has undertaken a minimum of 12 significant event reviews in the past 3y. which could include (if these have occurred) new cancer diagnoses	Total of 4 points for 12 significant event reviews	

Guidelines for urgent referral if suspected lung cancer[N]

Acute admission:
* Stridor
* Superior vena cava obstruction (swelling of face/neck with fixed ↑ JVP)

Urgent referral to a team specializing in management of lung cancer

* Persistent haemoptysis (in smokers/ex-smokers aged ≥40y.
* CXR suggestive of lung cancer (including pleural effusion and slowly resolving consolidation)
* Normal CXR where there is high suspicion of lung cancer

* History of asbestos exposure and recent onset of chest pain, shortness of breath or unexplained systemic symptoms where a CXR indicates pleural effusion, pleural mass or any suspicious lung pathology

Urgent CXR

* Haemoptysis
* Any of the following if unexplained or present for more >3wk.:

  * Cough
  * Chest/shoulder pain
  * Dyspnoea
  * Weight loss
  * Chest signs
  * Hoarseness (refer urgently to ENT if CXR is normal)

  * Finger clubbing
  * Cervical or supraclavicular lymphadenopathy
  * Features suggestive of metastases from a lung cancer e.g. secondaries in the brain, bone, liver or skin

Advice for patients: Information and support for patients

Lung cancer resources directory 🖳 www.cancerindex.org
The Roy Castle Lung Cancer Foundation ☎ 0800 358 7200
🖳 www.roycastle.org
Cancerbacup ☎ 0808 800 1234 🖳 www.cancerbacup.org.uk
British Lung Foundation ☎ 08458 50 50 20
🖳 www.lunguk.org

Pneumothorax

Air in the pleural cavity (Figure 4.13). >½ cases are due to trauma of some kind – the rest are spontaneous. 2 peaks in incidence are seen – 3rd to 4th decade and 8th to 9th decade.

Tension pneumothorax

- Complication of traumatic pneumothorax; rare after spontaneous pneumothorax.
- A valvular mechanism develops – air is sucked into the pleural space during inspiration but cannot be expelled during expiration. The pressure within the pleural space ↑, the lung deflates further, the mediastinum shifts to the opposite side of the chest and venous return ↓.
- Can be rapidly fatal.

Clinical features:

- Agitated and distressed patient often with a history of chest trauma
- Tachycardia
- Sweating
- Signs of a large pneumothorax – ↓ breath sounds and ↓ chest movement on the affected side
- Mediastinal shift – trachea deviated away from the side of the pneumothorax

> ### Action
> #### If suspected
> - Sit the patient upright if possible
> - Insert a large-bore cannula through the 2nd intercostal space of the chest wall in the mid-clavicular line on the side of the pneumothorax to relieve the pressure in the pleural space
> - Transfer as an emergency to hospital.

Spontaneous pneumothorax

Risk factors:

- Previous pneumothorax
- Smoking
- Ascent in an aeroplane
- Diving

Cause:

- **In patients <40y.:** Usually due to rupture of a pleural bleb. Typical patient is tall, thin and male (♂:♀ ≈ 6:1)
- **Patients >40y.:** Usually due to COPD (70–80%)
- **Rarer causes:** Asthma, pneumonia, TB, lung cancer, pulmonary fibrosis

Presentation:

- Sudden onset of pleuritic chest pain or ↑ breathlessness ± pallor and tachycardia.
- *Examination:* Look for resonant percussion note, ↓ or absent breath sounds – signs may be absent if the pneumothorax is small.

Management:

- Refer for CXR.
- If pneumothorax is confirmed, seek specialist advice about further management.

- Small pneumothoraces usually resolve spontaneously (50% collapse takes ~40d. to resorb) – monitor until completely resolved.
- Larger pneumothoraces may require admission for aspiration or a chest drain.
- Smoking cessation ↓ risk of recurrence.

Traumatic pneumothorax: Trauma may not initially be obvious – ask about injections around the chest area e.g. acupuncture (to neck and shoulders as well as chest); aspiration of breast lump etc.

Presentation and management: As for spontaneous pneumothorax (opposite).

Further information

British Thoracic Society Guidelines for the management of spontaneous pneumothorax (2003) ▢ www.brit-thoracic.org.uk

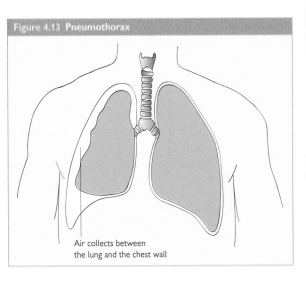

Figure 4.13 Pneumothorax

Air collects between the lung and the chest wall

Pulmonary embolism

Venous thrombi – usually from a deep vein thrombosis in the leg – pass into the pulmonary circulation and block blood flow to the lungs. Without treatment 20% with proximal deep vein thrombosis develop pulmonary embolus (PE). Fatal in ~1:10 cases causing ~20,000 deaths/y. in UK hospitals.

Risk factors
- Immobility – long flight or bus journey, post-op, plaster cast
- Smoking
- COC pill
- Pregnancy or puerperium
- Malignancy
- Past history or family history of DVT or PE

Presentation
Symptoms: Acute dyspnoea, pleuritic chest pain, haemoptysis, syncope. Large clots can be rapidly fatal.

Signs
- Hypotension
- Tachycardia
- Cyanosis
- Tachypnoea
- Pleural rub
- ↑JVP

Look for a source of emboli, though often DVT is not clinically obvious.

🛈 Recurrent small emboli can cause pulmonary hypertension (📖 p.140).

⚠ Have a high level of suspicion. Patients may have minimal symptoms/signs apart from some pleuritis pain and dyspnoea. PE in the community can be linked with surgical procedures done 2–3wk. previously.

Differential diagnosis
- Pneumonia and pleurisy
- MI/unstable angina
- Other causes of acute breathlessness – acute LVF, asthma, exacerbation of COPD, pneumothorax, shock (e.g. due to anaphylaxis), arrhythmia, hyperventilation
- Other causes of acute chest pain – aortic dissection, rib fracture, musculoskeletal chest pain, pericarditis, oesophageal spasm, shingles

Immediate action: If suspected, give oxygen as soon as possible and admit as an acute medical emergency.

Specialist management
- Involves investigation to prove diagnosis (ventilation-perfusion (VQ) scan, CT and/or pulmonary angiography).
- Thrombolytic therapy is controversial but usually given for major (life-threatening) PEs.
- In all cases of proven PE, anticoagulation is started in hospital or by a hospital-at-home service before discharge to general practice. Warfarin should be continued for 6mo. Aim to keep the INR ≈2.5 (range 2–3).

Thromboembolism in pregnancy[G]: Commonest direct cause of maternal death in the UK. Pregnancy ↑ risk of thromboembolism x 10. Incidence ≈ 1:100 pregnancies (20–50% antenatal).

Major risk factors: Age >35y; obesity – BMI >30kg/m^2

Other risk factors
- *Obstetric history* – parity >4, prolonged bed rest/immobility, dehydration (e.g. hyperemesis, ovarian hyperstimulation), severe infection (e.g. pyelonephritis), pre-eclampsia, prolonged labour, Caesarian section, high instrumental delivery, any other surgical procedure in pregnancy or the puerperium.
- *Family history* – venous thromboembolism
- *Medical history* – thromboembolism, thrombophilia, gross varicose veins, sickle cell disease, myeloproliferative disorders, inflammatory disorders (e.g. inflammatory bowel disease), nephritic syndrome, certain cardiac conditions
- *Other* – smoker

Management: Warfarin is teratogenic when used in the 1st trimester of pregnancy and can ↑ miscarriage, maternal and foetal haemorrhage, and stillbirth rates. Avoid during pregnancy. Warfarin is safe post-partum and during breast-feeding. Low molecular weight heparin (LMWH) is a safe alternative. Refer for expert advice.

Prevention: Ideally screen all women with a past history of thromboembolism for thrombophilia prior to conception. Prophylaxis is required if a patient has a thrombophilia or past history of pregnancy or COC-associated thromboembolism. LMWH is used antenatally and for up to 6wk. post-partum - refer for expert advice.

Antiphospholipid syndrome: Antiphospholipid antibodies (lupus anticoagulant and/or anticardiolipin antibodies) and a history of ≥1 of:
- arterial thrombosis
- venous thrombosis
- recurrent pregnancy loss (typically 2nd trimester).

Can be 1° (occurs alone) or 2° to another connective tissue disease – usually systemic lupus erythematosis.

Associated with
- ↑ risk of thrombosis
- ↑ risk of pre-eclampsia
- ↑ pregnancy loss – causes ~20% of recurrent miscarriages; <20% pregnancies result in live birth.

Management: Specialist referral is essential. Treatment is with aspirin and LMWH from 6–34wk.

Further information
Royal College of Obstetricians and Gynaecologists
🖳 www.rcog.org.uk
- Thromboprophylaxis during pregnancy, labour and after vaginal delivery (2004)
- Thromboembolic disease in pregnancy and the puerperium (2001)

Heparin in the community: Only use on specialist advice. Usually s/cut LMWH used as it does not need daily monitoring.

Warfarin: Acts by antagonizing the effects of vitamin K and thus ↓ clotting tendency. It takes 48–72h. for anticoagulant effect to develop fully, so for pulmonary embolus acute anticoagulation is with heparin in hospital and the patient is discharged on warfarin once the INR is in the therapeutic range. Indications and target INRs – Table 4.11.

Monitoring: Table 4.12. If there is a change in clinical state monitor more frequently until steady state is re-established. Have an explicit system for handling results promptly, making informed decisions on further treatment and testing, and communicating results to patients. Monitor the process with regular audit.

> ⚠ Warfarin is a dangerous drug:
> • It causes numerous admissions every year with bleeding
> • It interacts with a large number of drugs, including aspirin, some antibiotics, cimetidine, corticosteroids, and NSAIDs.
> • It is teratogenic.

Recurrent arterial thrombosis/embolism on anticoagulants
Seek specialist advice. *Consider:*
• Compliance
• Modifiable risk factors – smoking, ↑ BP, lipids
• Cardiac sources of emboli (echo)
• Thrombophilias
• Arteritis e.g. collagen disorders, syphilis
• Malignant disease.

Further information
SIGN Antithrombotic therapy (1999) 🖳 www.sign.ac.uk
British Journal of Haematology Guidelines on oral anticoagulation (3rd edition – 1999) **101**: 374–87 🖳 www.bcshguidelines.com

Table 4.11 Indications for oral anticoagulation and target INR		
Indication	Target INR (target range)	Duration of treatment
1st PE/proximal vein thrombosis and no persistent risk factors	2.5 (2.0–3.0)	6mo.
Prophylaxis of recurrent DVT/PE		
occurring on warfarin *occurring off warfarin*	3.5 (3.0–4.0) 2.5 (2.0–3.0)	Long term
Inherited thrombophilia with previous episode of thrombosis	2.5 (2.0–3.0)	Long term
Antiphospholipid syndrome	2.5–3.5	Long term

Table 4.12 Warfarin therapy: recall periods during maintenance therapy

INR	Recall interval and action
1 INR high ⚠ If INR>8 – admit	Recall 7–14d. Stop treatment for 1–3d. (max 1wk. in prosthetic valve patients) and restart at a lower dose.
1 INR low	↑ dose and recall in 7–14d.
1 therapeutic INR	Recall 4wk.
2 therapeutic INRs	Recall 6wk. (maximum interval if prosthetic heart valve).
3 therapeutic INRs	Recall 8wk.*
4 therapeutic INRs	Recall 10wk.*
5 therapeutic INRs	Recall 12wk.*

* Except prosthetic heart valves where maximum recall interval is 6wk.

GMS contract

Records 9	For repeat medicines, an indication for the drug can be identified in the records (for drugs added to the repeat prescription with effect from 1.4.2004)	4 points	Minimum standard 80%

Anticoagulation monitoring may be provided by practices as a national enhanced service – 📖 p.248

Diffuse parenchymal lung diseases

Also known as interstitial lung disease or diffuse lung disease. Comprises over 200 different diseases (many rare) in which inflammation affects the alveolar wall, leading to fluid in the alveolar air spaces.

Presentation: Diffuse shadowing on CXR (may be an incidental finding) ± increasing dyspnoea ± cough.

Assessment
History:
- Careful history of occupational and environmental exposure to allergens e.g. occupational dust exposure, pets (especially birds).
- Past/present medical history and family history – particularly looking for history of or suggesting systemic disease and/or immunosuppression.
- Drug and smoking history.
- Travel.

Examination
- Full examination looking for evidence of systemic disease e.g. fever, rashes or other skin changes, eye signs (particularly red eye), hepatomegaly and/or splenomegaly, arthritis.
- Respiratory examination.

Investigations: As well as CXR, consider:
- **Blood:** FBC, ESR, liver and kidney function tests, thyroid function tests, autoimmune profile
- **Lung function tests:** Usually show restrictive picture (Figure 4.14) – rarely no abnormalities or obstructive picture.

Classification: Table 4.13

Hypersensitivity pneumonitis: *(farmer's lung; bird fancier's lung)* Formerly known as extrinsic allergic alveolitis. Inhaled particles (e.g. fungal spores or avian proteins) provoke an allergic reaction in the lungs of hypersensitive individuals.

Presentation: Both may occur together:
- **Acute reaction:** 2–4h. post-exposure. Fever, malaise, dry cough, shortness of breath.
- **Chronic reaction:** Malaise, weight ↓, exertional dyspnoea, fine crepitations in both lung fields.

Investigations
- **FBC:** ↑ neutrophils (acute reaction)
- **ESR** ↑ (acute reaction)
- **CXR** may be normal or show typical changes (shadowing, widespread small nodules or ground glass appearance)
- Diagnosis is based on history and high resolution CT scan findings. Serum precipitins to the provoking factor are found in ≥90%.

Management: If possible prevent further exposure to the allergen. Treatment is not usually required in acute attacks. Refer for advice on chronic management. If occupational exposure, may qualify as industrial disease and be eligible for compensation – 📖 p.224.

Table 4.13 Classification of diffuse parenchymal lung disease

Classification	Causes
Acute	Infective: • Bacterial (TB) • Viral (chickenpox, measles) • Fungal Allergy – drugs, fungi, helminths Toxins – drugs, gases Haemodynamic – LVF, fluid overload, renal failure Vasculitis Adult repiratory distress syndrome
Episodic	Eosinophilic pneumonia e.g. allergic bronchopulmonary aspergillosis Vasculitis e.g. Churg-Strauss syndrome Extrinsic allergic alveolitis Cryptogenic organizing pneumonia
Chronic due to occupational or environmental exposure	Dust induced – asbestosis, silicosis, coal worker's pneumoconiosis, siderosis (iron) – 📖 p.182 Farmer's lung Bird fancier's lung Radiation Drugs e.g. nitrofurantoin, sulphasalazine, gold, penicillamine, aspirin, amiodarone, bleomycin, methotrexate, hydralazine, heroin, methadone, oxygen
Chronic with evidence of systemic disease	Connective tissue disease e.g. RA, Sjögren's syndrome, SLE Neoplastic e.g. lymphoma Vasculitis e.g. Wegener's granulomatosis, Goodpasture's syndrome Sarcoidodis Inherited disorders e.g. tuberose sclerosis, neurofibromatosis Miscellaneous e.g. HIV, inflammatory bowel disease, post-bone marrow transplant, amyloidosis
Chronic without evidence of systemic disease	Cryptogenic fibrosing alveolitis Chronic aspiration

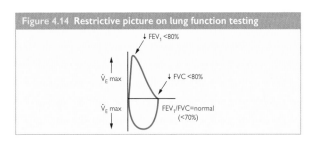

Figure 4.14 Restrictive picture on lung function testing

$\dot{V}_E$ max

↓ FEV$_1$ <80%

↓ FVC <80%

FEV$_1$/FVC=normal (<70%)

Fibrosing alveolitis: Incidence ↑ with age. May be:

Associated with other diseases:
- Connective tissue disease (33%)
- Chronic active hepatitis
- Renal tubular acidosis
- Autoimmune thyroid disease
- Ulcerative colitis

Associated with drug use:
- Cytotoxics e.g. busulphan, bleomycin, methotrexate
- Cardiac drugs e.g. amiodarone
- Antibiotics e.g. nitrofurantoin
- Analgesics e.g. diamorphine
- Rheumatological drugs e.g. gold, penicillamine
- Poisons e.g. paraquat

Idiopathic ('cryptogenic fibrosing alveolitis'): Occupational exposure to wood or metal dust may be implicated.

Presentation
- Progressive exertional dyspnoea and dry cough
- Clubbing (>50%)
- Fine end-inspiratory crepitations
- Malaise
- Weight ↓

In advanced cases: Central cyanosis and right heart failure.

CXR: Diffuse shadowing.

Lung function tests: Restrictive picture.

Differential diagnosis
- LVF
- COPD
- Other causes of lung fibrosis – dust exposure (coal, asbestos, silica, farmer's lung, bird fancier's lung)
- Inhalant exposure (O_2, Nitrous dioxide)
- Drugs
- Radiation

Management: Refer to a respiratory physician – if due to industrial exposure may be classified as an industrial disease and qualify for compensation (📖 p.224) Treatment is with oral steroids ± immunosuppressants. Lung transplant is a last option. 5y. survival is <50% but can be very variable. (range 1–20y.).

Sarcoidosis: Multisystem inflammatory disease of unknown cause characterized by non-caseating granulomata. May affect any organ and patients of any age but typically presents with lung granulomata in a young adult. ♀>♂.

Presentation
30–50% patients are asymptomatic and diagnosed on CXR done for other reasons.

Acute sarcoidosis (Löfgren's syndrome)
- Polyarthralgia
- Swinging fever
- Erythema nodosum
- Bilateral hilar lymphadenopathy on CXR

Insidious onset: CXR shows hilar lymphadenopathy – may be an incidental finding. If symptomatic, usually presents with tiredness, malaise, weight loss and/or arthralgia. 15% have lung symptoms with gradual onset of progressive exertional dyspnoea and dry cough.

Non-respiratory manifestations of sarcoidosis:
- Fever and malaise
- Erythema nodosum
- Lupus pernio (blue–red nodules on the nose, face and/or hands)
- Scar infiltration
- Enlarged lacrimal glands
- Hypopyon
- Uveitis
- Arthralgia
- Arrhythmias
- Heart failure
- Pericardial effusion
- Cranial and/or peripheral nerve palsies
- Seizures
- Hypercalcaemia
- Renal stones
- Lymphadenopathy
- Hepatosplenomegaly

Management: Refer any patient with bilateral hilar lymphadenopathy for further investigation. Steroids are widely used to treat sarcoidosis (± azathioprine, methotrexate or chloroquine) – relapse is common following withdrawal of treatment.

Prognosis:
- Remits without treatment in 2 out of 3 cases. ~30% have chronic progressive disease.
- Acute sarcoidosis has a particularly good prognosis with the majority resolving within 1–2y.
- Mortality is <3% – usually death is due to CCF and/or cor pulmonale.

Occupational lung disease: 📖 p.182

Further information
British Thoracic Society The diagnosis, assessment and treatment of diffuse parenchymal lung disease in adults *Thorax* (1999) 54 (Suppl 1) 🖥 www.brit-thoracic.org.uk

181

Occupational lung disease

Exposure to gases, vapours and dusts at work can lead to lung disease.

Coal worker's pneumoconiosis: 90% of all compensated industrial lung disease in the UK. 'Pneumoconiosis' means accumulation of dust in the lungs and tissue reaction to its presence. Incidence is related to total dust exposure. Divides into:

- *Simple pneumoconiosis:* Deposition of coal dust in the lung. Graded on CXR appearance. Grading determines whether disability benefit is payable in the UK. Effect on lung function is debated. Predisposes to progressive massive fibrosis (below).
- *Progressive massive fibrosis:* Round fibrotic masses several cm diameter form in the upper lobes. Presents with exertional dyspnoea, cough, black sputum and eventually respiratory failure. Symptoms progress (or may even start) after exposure to coal dust has ceased. Lung function tests show a mixed restrictive and obstructive picture with loss of lung volume, irreversible airflow limitation and ↓ gas transfer.

Asbestosis: Before legislation banning its use, exposure was widespread and occurred particularly in naval shipyards and power stations. Effects of asbestos exposure – Table 4.14. Consider diagnosis in relatives who came into contact with asbestos whilst washing clothes etc. too. Deaths from mesothelioma are increasing and likely to peak in 2020.

Silicosis: Uncommon. Affects stonemasons, pottery workers, workers exposed to sand-blasting and fettlers (remove sand from metal casts). Caused by inhalation of silica. CXR appearance is distinctive. Presents with exertional dyspnoea ± cough. *Lung function tests:* As for progressive massive fibrosis (above). Associated with ↑ risk of lung cancer and TB.

Byssinosis: Affects cotton mill workers. Symptoms (tightness in the chest, cough and breathlessness) start on the 1st day back at work after a break (Monday sickness) with improvement as the week progresses. CXR is normal.

Berylliosis: Rare. Long latent period. Affects workers in the aerospace, nuclear power and electrical industries and their close relatives. Presents similarly to sarcoidosis (📖 p.180).

Iron (siderosis), barium (baritosis) and tin (stannosis) dust inhalation: Result in dramatic dense nodular shadowing on the CXR but effects on lung function and symptoms are often minimal.

Occupational asthma: >200 industrial materials cause occupational asthma. Important causes are recognized occupational diseases in the UK – patients may be eligible for statutory compensation if they apply <10y. after leaving the occupation in which asthma developed. Suspect if a patient has symptoms which improve on days away from work/holiday.

Extrinsic allergic alveolitis ('farmer's lung') – 📖 p.178

Management: In all cases refer to a respiratory physician for confirmation of diagnosis (essential if seeking compensation) and advice on management.

Table 4.14 Conditions caused by asbestos exposure

Condition	Asbestos exposure	Features/management
Benign pleural effusion	Usually occurs <20y. after exposure	Increasing dyspnoea ± pleuritic pain. Refer for drainage of effusion. May be recurrent and require pleurodesis.
Bilateral diffuse pleural thickening*	Follows light or moderate exposure to asbestos May progress even in the absence of further exposure	Defined as pleural thickening >5mm thick covering >¼ of the chest wall. Symptoms: exertional dyspnoea. Lung function tests: restrictive picture. Treatment is symptomatic.
Asbestosis*	Follows heavy exposure after a 5–10y. interval	Presents with progressive dyspnoea, finger clubbing and basal end-expiratory crackles. CXR: 'honeycomb lung' – diffuse streaky shadowing. Lung function tests: severe restrictive defect and ↓ gas transfer. Treatment is symptomatic.
Mesothelioma*	Can follow even light exposure to asbestos 20–40y. time lag between exposure and appearance of disease	Presents with increasing shortness of breath ± pleuritic pain. Examination and CXR reveal unilateral (rarely bilateral) effusion. There is no effective active treatment. Palliative care – 📖 p.190. Median survival is 2y. from diagnosis.
Asbestosis-related lung cancer*	Patients exposed to asbestos who have evidence of that exposure (pleural plaques, bilateral pleural thickening or asbestosis) have an ↑ risk of bronchial carcinoma – usually adenocarcinoma. Smokers exposed to asbestos have a 5x ↑ risk compared to non-smokers exposed to asbestos. Manage as for lung cancer – 📖 p.170.	

* Eligible for industrial injuries benefit in the UK.

183

GP Notes

Advice for patients: Advise patients they may be entitled to compensation and/or benefits if they suffer from an occupational lung disease. Relatives exposed to asbestos e.g. through washing workers' clothes may be elligible for compensation too.

Industrial disease reporting and compensation: 📖 p.224

Benefits: 📖 pp.210–21

Advice for patients: Information and support for patients

British Lung Foundation ☎ 08458 50 50 20 🖥 www.lunguk.org

Snoring and obstructive sleep apnoea

Snoring: During sleep, the pharyngeal airway narrows due to ↑ dilator muscle tone. Snoring is vibratory noise generated from the pharynx and soft palate as air passes through the narrowed space. Further narrowing produces louder snoring, laboured inspiration and eventually episodic apnoea. Social consequences are the usual reason for patients to seek help: banishment from the bedroom, marital disharmony, no holidays, fear of travelling or falling asleep in a public place etc.

Obstructive sleep apnoea: Occurs when the pharyngeal airway completely closes during sleep → apnoeic episodes. ↑ inspiratory effort is sensed by the brain and a transient arousal provoked. A few of these arousals don't matter, but many (sometimes hundreds) per night → fragmented sleep and consequent daytime sleepiness.

Clinical features
- **Dominant features:** Excessive daytime sleepiness (not tiredness – Epworth Sleepiness Scale is a useful assessment tool – see opposite), impaired concentration, snoring
- **Other features:** Unrefreshing sleep, choking episodes during sleep, witnessed apnoeic episodes, restless sleep, irritability/personality change, nocturia, ↓ libido

Causes of snoring and sleep apnoea
- Overweight (neck circumference >16")
- Nasal congestion
- Evening alcohol/sedatives
- Large tonsils
- Receding lower jaw
- Smoking
- Hypothyroidism
- Menopause

Sleep apnoea in children: (📖 p.97)

Management of snoring *without* sleep apnoea[G]
Initial approaches:
- Suggest changing sleeping position – discourage from sleeping on back e.g. by wearing a bra backwards with a tennis ball in it.
- Elevate head of the bed e.g. prop up on bricks – can ↓ nasal congestion.
- Limit pillows to 1 thick/2 thin pillows to maximize pharyngeal size.
- ↓ weight if obese.
- ↓ or stop evening alcohol/sleeping tablets.
- Suggest partner tries ear plugs – purchase from the chemist – takes several nights to get used to wearing them.

If clinically indicated:
- For nasal congestion – start beclometasone nasal spray (applied head downwards) 2 puffs bd ± ipratropium nasal spray 2 puffs nocte.
- Check TFTs to exclude hypothyroidism.
- Discuss the use of HRT in menopausal women.

If simple measures fail: Refer to:
- Dentist or ENT for a mandibular advancement device
- ENT for surgery – septal straightening, polypectomy, turbinate reduction, tonsillectomy or uvulopalatopharyngoplasty.

Management of sleep apnoea[G]

- Advise patients to ↓ weight if obese.
- ↓ or stop evening alcohol/sleeping tablets.
- Refer to a sleep unit/physician with a special interest in sleep problems.
- If diagnosis of obstructive sleep apnoea is proven and causing significant daytime sleepiness, usual treatment is with CPAP therapy at night.
- Mandibular advancement devices are alternatives if patients can't tolerate CPAP or have mild symptoms with no daytime sleepiness.
- Occasionally, if large tonsils, referral to ENT for surgery if warranted.

The Epworth Sleepiness Scale

How likely are you to doze off or fall asleep in the following situations, in contrast to feeling just tired?

This refers to your usual way of life in recent times. Even if you have not done some of these things recently, try to work out how they would have affected you.

Situation	Chance of dozing
Sitting and reading	☐
Watching TV	☐
Sitting inactive in a public place (e.g. a theatre or a meeting)	☐
As a passenger in a car for an hour without a break	☐
Lying down to rest in the afternoon when circumstances permit	☐
Sitting and talking to someone	☐
Sitting quietly after a lunch without alcohol	☐
In a car, while stopped for a few minutes in traffic	☐
0 – No chance of dozing 2 – Moderate chance of dozing	
1 – Slight chance of dozing 3 – High chance of dozing	
Score > 10 – consider sleep apnoea	

185

GP Notes:

❶ Snoring may be used by the spouse as an excuse to leave the marital bed and may actually be trivial/absent. If suspected ask the patient to bring a cassette recording of the offending noise.

⚠ Patients who are sleepy in the day shouldn't drive. Once sleep apnoea is confirmed, they must inform their insurance companies and the DVLA.

Advice for patients: Information and support for patients

The Sleep Apnoea Trust (SATA) ☎ 01494 527772
🖥 www.sleep-apnoea-trust.org

Further information

SIGN/British Thoracic Society Management of obstructive sleep apnoea/ hypopnoea syndrome in adults (2003) 🖥 www.sign.ac.uk

The Epworth Sleepiness Scale © M.W. Jones, 1990–97, reproduced with permission.

Chronic disease management

The predominant disease pattern in the developed world is one of chronic or long-term illness. In the UK, 17.5 million adults are currently living with a chronic disease. Patients with all types of chronic lung disease are included in this group. Although details of chronic illness management depend on the illness, people with chronic diseases of all types have much in common with each other. *They all:*

- Have similar concerns and problems
- Must deal not only with their disease(s) but also the impact it has on their lives and emotions.

Common elements of effective chronic illness management

Involvement of the whole family: Chronic diseases do not only affect the patient but everyone in a family.

Collaboration between service providers and patients/ carers:
- Negotiate and agree a definition of the problem.
- Agree targets and goals for management.
- Develop an individualized self-management plan.

Personalized written care plan: Take into account patient/carers' views and experience and the current evidence base.

Tailored education in self-management: A patient with COPD or asthma spends ~3h./y. with a health professional – the other 8757h. he manages his own condition. Helping patients with chronic disease understand and take responsibility for their condition is imperative. User-led (i.e. led by someone who suffers from the condition) self-management education programmes are most effective and are becoming increasingly available.

Planned follow-up: Proactive follow-up according to the care plan – use of disease registers and call–recall systems is important.

Monitoring of outcome and adherence to treatment:
- Use of disease and treatment markers
- Monitoring of compliance e.g. checking prescription frequency
- Medicine management programmes

Tools and protocols for stepped care:
- Provide a framework for using limited resources to greatest effect.
- Start with limited professional input and systematic monitoring.
- Augment care for patients who do not achieve an acceptable outcome.
- Initial and subsequent treatments are selected according to evidence-based guidelines in light of a patient's progress.

Targeted use of specialist services: For those patients who cannot be managed in primary care alone.

Monitoring of process: Continually monitor management of patients with chronic disease through clinical governance mechanisms. Ensure changes are made promptly to optimize care.

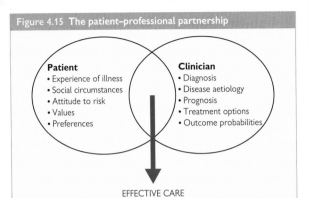

Figure 4.15 The patient–professional partnership

Patient
- Experience of illness
- Social circumstances
- Attitude to risk
- Values
- Preferences

Clinician
- Diagnosis
- Disease aetiology
- Prognosis
- Treatment options
- Outcome probabilities

EFFECTIVE CARE

GP Notes:

Common patient concerns may include
- Finding and using health services
- Finding and using other community resources
- Knowing how to recognize and respond to changes in a chronic disease
- Dealing with problems and emergencies
- Making decisions about when to seek medical help
- Using medicines and treatments effectively
- Knowing how to manage stress and depression that accompany a chronic illness
- Coping with fatigue, pain and sleep problems
- Getting enough exercise
- Maintaining good nutrition
- Working with your doctor(s) and other care providers
- Talking about your illness with family and friends
- Managing work, family and social activities

Expert patient schemes: Aim to train people with long-term chronic conditions e.g. asthma to 'self-manage' their condition more effectively on a day-to-day basis. 6wk. courses led by an 'expert patient' rather than health professional: topics covered are generic not disease-specific e.g. medicines management. Each week participants attend a 2½ h. session in groups of ~13. Also available on-line.

Further information
BMJ Von Korff *et al.* Organizing care for chronic illness (2002) **325**: 92–4 🖳 www.bmj.com
Expert Patient Scheme 🖳 www.expertpatients.nhs.uk

Rehabilitation

'Use strengthens, disuse debilitates'
Hippocrates (460–357 BC)

13–14% of the population have some disability. This is increasing as populations age and people survive longer with disability. Most patients are best managed by a multidisciplinary team in their home environment (if practicable) with a problem-oriented approach. Good interdisciplinary communication and coordination is essential and many patients benefit from specialist rehabilitation services. Psychological and sociocultural aspects are as important as medical aspects.

Principles of rehabilitation

- *Use of assessments/measures:* Central to management of any disability. Use validated measures accepted by all team members. Reassess regularly.
- *Teamwork:* Good outcomes are associated with clinicians working as a team towards a common goal with patients and their families (or carers) included as team members.
- *Goal setting:* Goals must be meaningful, challenging but achievable. Use short- and long-term goals. Involve the patient ± carer(s). Regularly renew, review and adapt.
- *Underlying approach to therapy:* All approaches focus on modification of impairment and improvement in function within everyday activities. Patients derive benefit from therapy focused on the management of disability.
- *Intensity/duration of therapy:* How much therapy is needed? Is there a minimum threshold below which there is no benefit at all? Studies on well-organized services show it is rare for patients to receive >2h. therapy/d. No one knows what is ideal.

Role of the GP

- The GP of any patient receiving rehabilitation in the community is a team member and may be the key worker who coordinates care.
- Maintain an open-door policy and encourage patients and carers to seek help for problems early.
- Try to become familiar with a patient's disease, even if it is rare. It is impossible to plan care without knowledge of course and prognosis and an easy way to lose a patient's confidence if you appear ignorant of their condition.
- If progress is slower than expected, or stalls, consider other medical problems (e.g. anaemia, hypothyroidism, dementia), a neurological event, depression and communication problems (e.g. poor vision/hearing).
- Information alone can improve outcome.

Care of informal carers: 📕 p.222

Benefits: 📕 p.209

GP Notes: Checklist of areas to cover

- Can physical symptoms be improved?
- Can the psychological symptoms be improved (including self-esteem)?
- Can functioning within the home be improved? (aids and adaptations within the home, extra help)
- Can functioning in the community be improved? (mobility outside the home, work, social activities)
- Can the patient's or carer's financial state be improved? (benefits)
- Does the carer need more support? (voluntary and self-help organizations, social services)

Advice for patients: Information and support for patients and carers

Support organizations for the patient's condition (e.g. Asthma UK – 📖 p.258)

Department of Work and Pensions 🖳 www.dwp.gov.uk ☎ *Benefits enquiry line* 0800 882200; 0800 243355 (minicom facility); 0800 441144 (for help with form completion)

Citizens' Advice Bureau 🖳 www.adviceguide.org.uk

Age Concern ☎ 0800 00 99 66 🖳 www.ageconcern.org.uk

Help the Aged ☎ 0800 800 65 65 🖳 www.helptheaged.org.uk

Disabled Living Foundation Advice about equipment and appliances ☎ 0845 130 9177 🖳 www.dlf.org.uk

Age Concern Wide range of information and factsheets ☎ Information line 0800 00 99 66 🖳 www.ageconcern.org.uk

Royal Association for Disability and Rehabilitation (RADAR) ☎ 020 7250 3222 🖳 www.radar.org.uk

Disablement Information and Advice Line (DIAL) ☎ 01302 310123

Palliative care in general practice

'Any man's death diminishes me because I am involved in mankind'
Devotions Meditation 17, John Donne (1572–1631)

Palliative care starts when the emphasis changes from curing the patient and prolonging life to relieving symptoms and maintaining well-being or 'quality of life'. GPs have 1–2 patients with terminal disease at any time and get more personally involved with them than any others.

The problems arising are a complex mix of physical, psychological, social, cultural and spiritual factors involving both patients and carers. To respond adequately, good lines of communication and close multi-disciplinary teamwork is needed. Local palliative care teams are invaluable sources of advice and support and frequently produce booklets with advice on aspects of palliative care for GPs.

Weakness, fatigue and drowsiness: Almost a universal symptom.
Reversible causes:
- Drugs – opiates, benzodiazepines, steroids (proximal muscle weakness), diuretics (dehydration and biochemical abnormalities), antihypertensives (postural hypotension)
- Emotional problems – depression, anxiety, fear, apathy
- Hypercalcaemia
- Other biochemical abnormalities – DM, electrolyte disturbance, uraemia, liver disease, thyroid dysfunction
- Anaemia
- Poor nutrition
- Infection
- Prolonged bed rest
- Raised intracranial pressure (drowsiness only)

Management:
- Treat reversible causes.
- If drowsiness and fatigue persist consider a trial of dexamethasone 4–6mg/d. or antidepressant. Although steroids make muscle wasting worse they may improve general fatigue and improve mobility.
- Psychological support of patients and carers – empathy, explanation.
- Physical support – referral to physiotherapist, review of aids and appliances, review of home layout (possibly with referral to OT), review of home care arrangements.
- Advice on modification of lifestyle.

Further information
Hospice information ☎ 0870 903 3903
🖫 www.hospiceinformation.info
Woodruff & Doyle *The IAHPC Manual of Palliative Care* (2nd edn) (2004) IAHPC Press ISBN 0-9758525-1-5
🖫 www.hospicecare.com/manual/IAHPCmanual.htm

GMS contract		
Palliative Care 1	The practice has a complete register available of all patients in need of palliative care/support	3 points
Palliative Care 2	The practice has regular (at least every 3mo.) multidisciplinary case review meetings where all patients on the palliative care register are discussed	3 points

GP Notes: Basic rules of symptom control

Symptom control must be tailored to the needs of the individual.
- Carefully diagnose the cause of the symptom.
- Explain the symptom to the patient.
- Discuss treatment options.
- Set realistic goals.
- Anticipate likely problems.
- Review regularly.

⚠ Death is the natural end to life – not a failure of medicine.

Advice for patients: Advice and support for patients and their carers

Cancerbacup ☎ 0808 800 1234 🖥 www.cancerbacup.org.uk
Macmillan Cancer Relief ☎ 0808 808 2020
🖥 www.macmillan.org.uk

Pain control: Pain control is the cornerstone of palliative care. Cancer pain is multifactorial – be aware of physical and psychological factors. The majority of pain can be managed using a step-by-step approach to pain relief (Figure 4.16).

Step 1: Non-opioid
- Start treatment with paracetamol 1g every 4h. REGULARLY (maximum daily dose 4g).
- If this is not adequate in 24h., stop and either try a NSAID e.g. ibuprofen 400mg tds (if appropriate) alone or in combination with paracetamol, or proceed to step 2.

Step 2: Weak opioid + non-opioid
- Start treatment with a combined preparation of paracetamol with codeine or dihydrocodeine. Combining 2 analgesics with different mechanisms of action enables better pain control than using either drug alone at that dose.
- Combinations have ↓ dose-related side-effects but the range of side-effects is ↑ (additive effects of 2 drugs).
- Combinations using full-dose opiate (e.g. Solpadol™) are more effective than paracetamol alone but it is cheaper and more flexible if constituents are prescribed separately e.g. 'paracetamol 500mg/codeine 30mg'.
- Advise patients to take tablets regularly and not to assess efficacy after only a couple of doses.

  ⓘ There is no additional analgesic benefit from preparations which contain paracetamol + 8mg of codeine, as opposed to paracetamol alone.

Step 3: Strong opioid + non-opioid
- Use immediate-release morphine tablets or morphine solution, depending on patient preference. 2 tablets of co-codamol contain 60mg of codeine which is equi-analgesic to ~ 6mg of oral morphine. If changing to morphine, use a minimum dose of 5mg.
- Chronic pain may not respond to an opiate. Give for a 2wk. trial and only continue if of proven benefit. Worries of tolerance/addiction are unfounded for patients with true opioid-sensitive pain. If the pain seems responsive to opioids and there are no undue side-effects, ↑ the dose upwards by 30–50% every 24h. until pain is controlled.

  ⚠ Take care if the patient is elderly or in renal failure – consider starting with a ↓ dose of morphine.

Addition of co-analgesics and adjuvant drugs: In combination with analgesics, can enhance pain control. Examples include:
- *Antidepressants* – for nerve pain and depression associated with pain
- *Anticonvulsants* – neuropathic pain
- *Corticosteroids* – pain due to oedema
- *Muscle relaxants* – muscle cramp pain
- *Antispasmodics* – bowel colic
- *Antibiotics* – infection pain
- *Night sedative* – when lack of sleep is lowering pain threshold
- *Anxiolytic* – when anxiety is making pain worse (relaxation exercises may also help in these circumstances).

Figure 4.16 The World Health Organization analgesics ladder

Step 3

Severe pain
Strong opioids e.g. morphine, hydromorphone, diamorphine, fentanyl TTS patch

± non-opioid (paracetamol and/or NSAID)

Step 2

Moderate pain
Weak opioids e.g. tramadol, dihydrocodeine

± non-opioid (paracetamol and/or NSAID)

Step 1

Mild pain
Non-opioids e.g. NSAID and/or paracetamol

Co-analgesics: drugs, nerve blocks, TENS, relaxation, acupuncture

Specific therapies: surgery, physiotherapy

Address psychosocial problems

GP Notes:

Troubleshooting

- Continuing pain and frequent prn doses – ↑ regular dose.
- Persisting side-effects (drowsiness, jerking, vomiting, confusion) – ↓ regular dose.
- Considerable pain despite marked side-effects – use alternative.

Quick conversions

From	To	Conversion	Example
Oral morphine (total dose)	s/cut diamorphine	÷ by 3	60÷3 = 20mg diamorphine by syringe driver over 24h.
e.g. 10mg morphine 4 hourly = 60mg oral morphine in 24h.	s/cut morphine	÷ by 2	60÷2 = 30mg morphine by syringe driver over 24h.
	oral oxycodone	÷ by 2	60÷2 = 30mg oral oxycodone in divided doses over 24h.
	oral hydromorphone	÷ by 7.5	60÷7.5 = (60×2)÷15 = 8mg hydromorphone in divided doses over 24h.

🛈 If total 24h. dose is equivalent to 360mg morphine or more – get specialist advice.

Bone pain: Metastases to bone are common with lung cancers.
- Try NSAIDs.
- Consider referral for palliative radiotherapy, strontium treatment (prostate cancer) or IV bisphosphonates (↓ pain in myeloma, breast and prostate cancer).
- Refer to orthopaedics if any lytic metastases at risk of fracture for consideration of pinning.

Figure 4.16 is reproduced with permission from the World Health Organization 🖥 www.who.int

Stridor and cough in terminal care

Stridor: Coarse wheezing sound that results from the obstruction of a major airway e.g. larynx.

Management:
- Corticosteroids (e.g. dexamethasone 16mg/d.) can give relief.
- Consider referral for radiotherapy or endoscopic insertion of a stent if appropriate.

If a terminal event: Sedate with high doses of midazolam (10–40mg repeated prn).

Cough: Troublesome symptom. Prolonged bouts of coughing are exhausting and frightening, especially if associated with breathlessness and/or haemoptysis.

Reversible causes: Box 4.7

Management

General measures
- Exclude any treatable cause for cough (e.g. ACE inhibitors).
- Advise upright body position.
- Steam inhalations, inhalations with menthol or tinct. Benz. Co (Friar's balsam) or nebulized saline can help.
- Refer for chest physiotherapy, relaxation and breathing control exercises if tolerated.
- Simple linctus 5–10ml prn can be helpful for dry cough. If not, consider low-dose opioid e.g. pholcodine 10ml tds, codeine linctus 30mg qds, Oramorph 5mg every 4h. or diamorphine 5–10mg/24h. via syringe driver. If already on opioids ↑ dose by 25%. Titrate dose until symptoms are controlled or side-effects.
- Diazepam 2–10mg tds can relieve anxiety and act as a central cough depressant simultaneously.

Specific measures:
- *Chest infection* – treat with nebulized saline to make secretions less viscous ± antibiotics (if not considered a terminal event).
- *Tumour* – consider referral for radiotherapy.
- *Post-nasal drip* – steam inhalations, steroid nasal spray or drops ± antibiotics.
- *Laryngeal irritation* – try inhaled steroids.
- *Bronchospasm* – try bronchodilators ± inhaled or oral steroids.
  🛈 Salbutamol may help cough even in the absence of wheeze.
- *Gastric reflux* – try antacids containing dimethicone (Gaviscon™, Asilone™).
- *Lung cancer* – try inhaled sodium cromoglycate 10mg qds; local anaesthesia using nebulized bupivacaine or lidocaine can be helpful – refer for specialist advice (avoid eating/drinking for 1h. afterwards to avoid aspiration). Palliative radiotherapy or chemotherapy can also relieve cough in patients with lung cancer – refer.
- ↓ *secretions* – try hyoscine 400–600mcgm 4–8 hourly (or 0.6–2.4mg/24h. via syringe driver) and/or ipratropium inhalers/nebulised ipratropium.

Box 4.7 **Reversible causes of cough**

- Infection
- Bronchospasm
- Gastro-oesophageal reflux
- Aspiration
- Drug induced e.g. ACE inhibitors
- Treatment related e.g. total body irradiation
- Malignant bronchial obstruction/ lung metastases
- Heart failure
- Secretions
- Pharyngeal candidiasis

Further information

BMJ Davis C ABC of palliative care: breathlessness, cough and other respiratory problems (1997) **315:** 931–4 ▢ www.bmj.com

Doyle *et al. Oxford Textbook of Palliative Medicine* (2005) Oxford University Press ISBN: 0198566980

Haemoptysis in terminal care

Expectoration of blood or blood-stained sputum. Bleeding due to cancer is most commonly from a primary carcinoma of the bronchus and a massive haemoptysis is usually from a squamous cell lung tumour lying centrally or causing cavitation.

Presentation

- Small episodes of haemoptysis occasionally herald a catastrophic bleed.
- Malaena rarely occurs in association with haemoptysis if enough blood is swallowed.
- Massive haemoptysis is rare but exceedingly distressing if it occurs.
- The patient is more likely to die from suffocation secondary to the bleed than from the bleed itself.

Management

Severe, life-threatening bleed: Make a decision whether the cause of the bleed is treatable or a terminal event. This is best done in advance but bleeding can't always be predicted.
- *Severe bleed – active treatment:* Briefly assess the severity of the bleed from history and examination. If a significant bleed is suspected:
  - Call for emergency ambulance support
  - Protect the airway
  - Lie the patient flat and lift legs higher than body (e.g. feet on pillow)
  - If the bleeding side is known, lie the patient on that side to protect the unaffected lung
  - Insert a large-bore IV cannula – the opportunity may be lost by the time the ambulance crew arrive. If possible take a sample for FBC and cross match on insertion
  - If available, give oxygen
  - If available, start plasma expander/IV fluids
  - Transfer as rapidly as possible to hospital.
- *Severe bleed – no active treatment:*
  - Stay with the patient.
  - Give sedative medication e.g. midazolam 20–40mg s/cut or IV or diazepam 10–20mg pr and diamorphine 5–10mg s/cut or IV.
  - Support carers as big bleeds are extremely distressing.

Non-life-threatening bleed: Reassure; monitor frequently.

Follow-up treatment: Follow-up is directed at cause if appropriate:
- Check FBC and clotting screen – if frequent bleeds or large bleed, on anticoagulants or possible bleeding tendency. Consider addressing clotting problem and/or iron supplements or transfusion
- Treat infection that might exacerbate a bleed
- Consider minimizing bleeding tendency with tranexamic acid 1g tds po – stop if no effect after 1wk. If effective continue for 1wk. after bleeding has stopped. Continue 500mg tds long-term if bleeding recurs and responds to a further course of treatment. Weigh up benefits of stopping bleeding against ↑ risk of stroke or MI

- Radiotherapy – consider referral if haemoptysis (not if multiple lung metastases), cutaneous bleeding or haematuria
- Referral for chemotherapy or palliative surgery e.g. cautery – options in some cases.

GP Notes:

🛈 In all patients likely to bleed, consider pre-warning carers and giving them a strategy. Risks of frightening a family with information about possible catastrophic haemoptysis need to be balanced against potential distress that could be caused by leaving a patient and family unprepared.

Breathlessness in terminal care

'Breathing is the greatest pleasure in life'
Giovanni Papini (1881–1956)

Breathlessness affects 70% of terminally ill patients. It is usually multi-factorial. Breathlessness always has a psychological element – being short of breath is frightening.

Causes: Figure 4.17

General management

Non-drug measures

- General reassurance
- Explanation of reasons for breathlessness and adaptations to lifestyle that might help
- Proper positioning – improved by sitting upright and straight
- Try a stream of air over the face e.g. fan, open window
- Breathing exercises can help – refer to physiotherapy. Exercises include diaphragmatic breathing and control of breathing rate; relaxation training/distraction training

Drug treatment

- Tenaceous secretions – try nebulized saline.
- Oral or subcutaneous opioids ↓ subjective sensation of breathlessness – start with 2.5mg Oramorph 4 hourly and titrate upwards.
- Try benzodiazepines – 2–5mg diazepam od/bd for background control and lorazepam 1–2mg sublingually prn in between.
- Oxygen has a variable effect and is worth a try.

Specific measures

- ***Airway compression, bronchoconstriction or lymphangitis:*** Consider referral for anti-cancer treatment. Otherwise try steroids (dexamethasone 4–8mg/d.).
- ***Intrinsic or extrinsic compression:*** Consider referral for radiotherapy, laser therapy or stenting.
- ***Pleural effusion:*** Consider referral for drainage ± pleuradesis.
- ***Pericardial effusion:*** Consider referral for aspiration in a cardiac unit
- ***Infection:*** Antibiotics ± physiotherapy – have a low threshold to treat with a broad-spectrum antibiotic if appropriate.
- ***Pneumothorax on CXR:*** Consider referral for chest drain.
- ***Ascites:*** Consider referral for paracentesis if causing breathlessness.
- ***Suspected pulmonary emboli:*** Consider anticoagulation – 📖 p.174.
- ***Wheeze:*** Try inhaled broncholdilators e.g. salbutamol inhaler.
- ***Excessive upper airway secretions:*** Try hyoscine 0.4–2.4mg/24h. or glycopyrronium 200–600mcgm/24h. (consult local palliative care team).
- ***Musculoskeletal pain*** can cause hypoventilation – treat with analgesia.
- ***Anaemia (Hb <10g/l):*** See opposite.
- ***Thick secretions:*** Consider referral for chest physiotherapy.
- ***Vocal cord palsy:*** Consider referral to ENT for teflon injection.

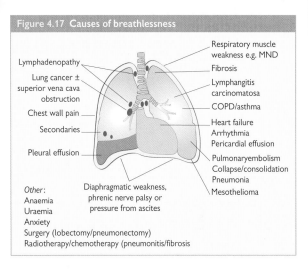

Figure 4.17 Causes of breathlessness

Lymphadenopathy

Lung cancer ± superior vena cava obstruction

Chest wall pain

Secondaries

Pleural effusion

Respiratory muscle weakness e.g. MND

Fibrosis

Lymphangitis carcinomatosa

COPD/asthma

Heart failure
Arrhythmia
Pericardial effusion

Pulmonary embolism
Collapse/consolidation
Pneumonia

Mesothelioma

Diaphragmatic weakness, phrenic nerve palsy or pressure from ascites

Other:
Anaemia
Uraemia
Anxiety
Surgery (lobectomy/pneumonectomy)
Radiotherapy/chemotherapy (pneumonitis/fibrosis)

Anaemia: Don't check for anaemia if there is no intention to transfuse.

● *If Hb <10g/dl and symptomatic:* Treat any reversible cause (e.g. iron deficiency, GI bleeding 2° to NSAIDs). Consider transfusion.
● *If transfused:* Record whether any benefit is derived (as, if not, further transfusions are futile) and the duration of benefit (if <3wk., repeat transfusions are impractical). Monitor for return of symptoms, repeat FBC and arrange repeat transfusion as needed.

Superior vena cava obstruction: 📖 p.200

Pulmonary embolus: 📖 p.174

Further information

BMJ Davis C ABC of palliative care: breathlessness, cough and other respiratory problems (1997) **315:** 931–4 🖥 www.bmj.com
Doyle et al. *Oxford Textbook Of Palliative Medicine* (2005) Oxford University Press ISBN: 0198566980

Emergencies in terminal care

Superior vena cava (SVC) obstruction: Due to infiltration of the vessel wall, clot within the superior vena cava or extrinsic pressure. 75% are due to 1° lung cancer (3% of patients with lung cancer have SVC obstruction). Lymphoma is the other major cause.

Presentation
- Shortness of breath/stridor
- Headache worse on stooping ± visual disturbances ± dizziness and collapse
- Swelling of the face, particularly around the eyes, neck, hands and arms, and/or injected cornea
- Examination: look for non-pulsatile distention of neck veins and dilated collateral veins (seen as small dilated veins over the anterior chest wall below the clavicles) in which blood courses downwards

Management
- Treat breathlessness (opiates – 5mg Oramorph™ 4 hourly ± benzodiazepine depending on the level of anxiety).
- Start corticosteroid (dexamethasone 16mg/d.).
- Refer urgently for oncology opinion. Palliative radiotherapy has a response rate of 70%. Stenting ± thrombolysis is also an option.

Raised intracranial pressure: Occurs with 1° or 2° brain tumours. Characterized by:
- Headache – worse on lying
- Vomiting
- Confusion
- Diplopia
- Convulsions
- Papilloedema

Management
- Unless a terminal event, refer patients urgently to neurosurgery for assessment. Options include insertion of a shunt/cranial radiotherapy.
- If no further active treatment is appropriate start symptomatic treatment – raise the head of the bed, start dexamethasone 16mg/d. (stop if no response in 1wk.), analgesia.

Bone fractures: Common in advanced disease due to osteoporosis, trauma as a result of falls, or metastases. Have a low index of suspicion if a new bony pain develops.

> ⚠ In the elderly, fracture of a long bone can present as acute confusion.

Management
- Analgesia
- Unless in a very terminal state, confirm the fracture on X-ray and refer to orthopaedics or radiotherapy urgently for consideration of fixation (long bones, wrist, neck of femur) and/or radiotherapy (rib fractures, vertebral fractures).

Spinal cord compression: Affects 5% of cancer patients – 70% in thoracic region. Presentation can be subtle. Maintain a *high* level of suspicion in all cancer patients who complain of back pain, especially those with known bony metastases or tumours likely to metastasize to bone.

Presentation
- Often back pain, worse on movement, appears before neurology.
- Neurological symptoms/signs can be non-specific – constipation, weak legs, urinary hesitancy.
- Lesions above L1 (lower end of spinal cord) may produce upper motor neurone signs (e.g. ↑ tone & reflexes) and a sensory level.
- Lesions below L1 may produce lower motor neurone signs (↓ tone & reflexes) and peri-anal numbness (cauda equina syndrome).

Management: Prompt treatment (<24–48h. from 1st neurological symptoms) is needed if there is any hope of restoring function. Once paralysed, <5% walk again. Treat with oral dexamethasone 16mg/d. and refer urgently for assessment and surgery/radiotherapy unless in final stages of disease.

Hypercalcaemia: Most common with:
- Myeloma (>30%)
- Breast cancer (40%) and
- Squamous cell cancers.

Presentation: Symptoms are non-specific:
- Thirst
- Polyuria and polydipsia
- Constipation
- Nausea and vomiting
- Abdominal pain
- ↓ appetite
- Depression
- Fatigue
- Confusion

⚠ Always suspect hypercalcaemia if someone is more ill than expected for no obvious reason. Untreated hypercalcaemia can be fatal.

Management: Depending on the general state of the patient, make a decision whether to treat the hypercalcaemia or not. If a decision is made *not* to treat, provide symptom control and don't check the serum calcium again. Active treatment depends on the level of symptoms and hypercalcaemia.

Asymptomatic patient with corrected calcium <3mmol/l: Monitor.

Symptomatic and/or corrected calcium >3mmol/l:
- Arrange treatment with pamidronate via oncologist/palliative care team immediately.
- Check serum calcium 7–10d. post-treatment. 20% do not respond and there is no benefit from retreating them.
- Effect of pamidronate lasts 20–30d. Consider maintenance with oral bisphosphonates (e.g. sodium clodronate) started 1wk. after the initial IV pamidronate or regular IV pamidronate. Many initially responsive to bisphosphonates become unresponsive with time.

The last 48 hours

It is notoriously difficult to predict when death will occur. Avoid the trap of predicting or making a guess unless absolutely pushed to do so. Talk in terms of 'days' or 'weeks'. For example:

'When we see someone deteriorating from week to week we are often talking in terms of weeks; when that deterioration is from day to day then we are usually talking in terms of days, but everyone is different.'

Symptoms and signs of death approaching
- Day by day deterioration
- Gaunt appearance
- Profound weakness – needs assistance with all care, may be bed-bound
- Difficulty swallowing medicines
- ↓ intake of food and fluids
- Drowsy or ↓ cognition – often unable to cooperate with carers

Goals of treatment in the last 48h.
- Ensure patients are comfortable – physically, emotionally and spiritually.
- Make the end of life peaceful and dignified; what is dignified for one patient may not be for another – ask.
- Support patients and carers so that the experience of death for those left behind is as positive as it can be.

Patients' wishes: Dying is a unique and special event for each individual. Helping to explore a patient's wishes about death and dying should not be a discussion left to the last 24h.

Advance directives/living wills: 📖 p.235

Different cultures: Different religious and cultural groups have different approaches to the dying process. It is important to be sensitive to cultural and religious beliefs. If in doubt ask a family member. You are more likely to cause offence by not asking than by asking.

Assessment of a patient's needs: Try to discover which problems are causing the patient/carers most concern and address those concerns where possible. Patients often under-report their symptoms and families/carers may misinterpret symptoms.

Physical examination: Keep examination to a minimum to avoid unnecessary interference. Check:
- Sites of discomfort/pain suggested by history or non-verbal cues
- Mouth
- Bladder and bowel.

Psychological assessment: Find out what the patient wants to know. Gently assessing how the patient feels about their disease and situation can shed light on their needs and distress.

Investigations: Any investigation at the end of life should have a clear and justifiable purpose (e.g. excluding a reversible condition where treatment would make the patient more comfortable). The need for investigations in the terminal stage of illness is minimal.

GP Notes: Talking about death and dying

Death is a taboo subject and few people feel comfortable discussing it, even though it is natural, certain, and happening all around us all the time.

Opening up discussion can be very liberating to patients who then may feel they are being given permission to talk about dying. Families do not like discussions about dying for fear that patients will 'give up'.

Sometimes the direct question 'Are you worried about dying?' is the most appropriate. Often patients' biggest fears are groundless and reassurance can be given. Where reassurance cannot be given it is helpful to break the fear down into constituent parts and try to sort out those aspects you can deal with.

Common fears
- *Fears associated with symptoms* e.g. pain will escalate to agony; breathing will stop if the patient falls asleep.
- *Emotional fears* e.g. increasing dependence on family. 'It would be better if I was out of the way.'
- *Past experience* e.g. past contact with patients who died with unpleasant symptoms.
- *Preferences about treatment or withholding treatment* e.g. 'What if nobody listens to me or takes my wishes seriously?'
- *Fears about morphine*
- *Death and dying* – fears of being dead and the process of dying need to be differentiated.

Review of medication
- Comfort is the priority. Stop unnecessary medication.
- Continue analgesia, anti-emetics, anxiolytics/antipsychotics and anticonvulsants.
- Diabetes can be managed with short-acting insulin as needed.
- Consider alternative routes of drug administration (e.g. syringe driver, patches).
- Explain changes to relatives/carers.

Symptom control: Dying patients tolerate symptoms very poorly because of their weakness. Nursing care is the mainstay of treatment. GPs do have a role though.
- Ensure new problems don't develop e.g. ensure use of appropriate mattresses and measures to prevent bed sores.
- Treat specific symptoms e.g. dry mouth.
- Think ahead – discuss treatment options which might be available later e.g. use of a syringe driver, buccal, pr or transcutaneous preparations to deliver medication when/if the oral route is no longer possible, use of strong analgesia which may also have a sedative effect.
- Ensure there is a clear management plan agreed between the medical and nursing team and the patient/family members. Anticipate probable needs of the patient so that immediate response can be made when the time comes – define clearly what should be done in the event of a symptom arising/worsening; ensure drugs or equipment that may be needed are in the home.

Referral to specialist palliative care services: Ideally involve specialist palliative care services before the terminal phase is reached. Referral in the terminal phase is appropriate when:
- One or more distressing symptoms prove difficult to control
- There is severe emotional distress
- There are dependent children and/or elderly vulnerable relatives involved.

Terminal anguish and spiritual distress
- Characterised by overwhelming distress
- Often related to unresolved conflict, guilt, fears or loss of control

Anxiety can be increased if
- Patients are unaware of the diagnosis, but feel people are lying to them
- They have certain symptoms such as breathlessness, haemorrhage and constant nausea or diarrhoea
- Weak religious conviction – convinced believers and convinced non-believers have less anxiety
- There are young dependent children or other dependent relatives
- Patients have unfinished business to attend to, such as legal affairs

Action: Empathic listening can itself be therapeutic. Talk to the patient, if possible, about dying and try to break down fears into component parts. Address those fears that can be dealt with. As a last resort, and after discussion with the patient (where possible) and/or relatives, consider sedation (see terminal restlessness/agitation).

Advice for patients: Patient experiences

Not wanting to be a burden
'I don't want to be a burden to my family, that is something that's definitely out of order as far as I'm concerned. I've seen other families that have endeavoured to cope with situations of that type when they couldn't and it practically destroyed the family.'

Choosing a place to die
'I go back to my wife who died from cancer. One of the things she said to me was, "I know I'm dying but I want to die in my own home." And my response was, "If we can manage to bring that wish to fulfilment we will do that." And with the help of my 2 daughters and the local community nurses and the doctor, we managed to achieve that. It was hard work. It was very emotional but we managed to carry out her last wish.'

'I think if the cancer got bad I would like to go to a hospice. My husband is not terribly practical when it comes to looking after someone who is very ill and I think that I would like, if it came to it, to be in a hospice where they control the pain for you and look after you.'

Worries about death and dying
'Again I don't know from the doctors what is likely to happen apart from they say I will just get weaker and weaker and as more pain occurs in the bones then I will be given more painkillers.'

'My biggest problem with thinking about death is not the actual dying because I can envisage that as going to sleep and not knowing anything about it, like you go in for surgery. You have the anaesthetic and you're gone and you know nothing about it and you just don't wake up. I think of death like that. What worries me is what's going to happen before, particularly with cancer because you hear so much about the pain. I've experienced pain, I've had the pain in this breast so I have experienced pain, and that side of it does worry me in wondering how I would cope with it.'

Acceptance of dying
'Everybody is so different. Some people can shout, some people can scream, some people are quiet, it's very different, difficult. But acceptance is a great thing. It heals the mind. You know, you didn't bring it on yourself. You didn't make yourself sick. It comes on. You don't know why. So, that's all I can say because that's all I can get from it. I accept it.'

'Life is a mixture of all sorts of things. There are sad moments, and there are moments when things have gone wrong, and there are moments when you can be upset and angry about things, but find the positives. And rejoice in those positives and rejoice in the life that you've had. Celebrate the life that you've had and come to terms with the fact that it will ultimately end. The only difference is that you now know and some people . . . well it comes to an end and they don't know about it.'

Patient experiences are reproduced with permission from the DIPEx patient experience database 🖳 www.dipex.org

205

Terminal restlessness: *Causes:*

- *Pain/discomfort* – urinary retention, constipation, pain which the patient cannot tell you about, excess secretions in throat
- *Opiate toxicity* – causes myoclonic jerking. The dose of morphine may need to be ↓ if a patient becomes uraemic
- *Biochemical causes* – ↑ Ca^{2+}, uraemia – ❗ if it has been decided not to treat abnormalities DON'T check for them
- *Psychological/spiritual distress.*

Management

- Treat reversible causes e.g. catheterization for retention, hyoscine to dry up secretions.
- If still restless, treat with a sedative. This does NOT shorten life but makes the patient and any relatives in attendance more comfortable.

Suitable drugs: Haloperidol 1–3mg tds po; chlorpromazine 25–50mg tds po; diazepam 2–10mg tds po, midazolam (10–100mg/24h. via syringe driver or 5mg stat) or levomepromazine (50–150mg/24h. via syringe driver or 6.25mg stat).

Excessive respiratory secretion (death rattle): Noisy, moist breathing. Rarely distresses patients but can be very distressing for relatives in attendance.

Management

- Reassure relatives that the patient is not suffering or choking.
- Try repositioning and/or tipping the bed head down (if possible) to reduce the noise.
- Treat prophylactically – it is easier to prevent secretions forming than remove accumulated secretions.

Suitable drugs

- Glycopyrronium – non-sedative – give 200mcgm/cut stat and review after 1h. If effective, give 200mcgm every 4h. by s/cut injection or 0.6–1.2mg/24h. via syringe driver.
- Hyoscine hydrobromide – sedative in high doses – give 400mcgm/cut stat and review response after 30min. If effective, give 400–600mcgm 4–8 hourly or 0.6–2.4mg/24h. via syringe driver. If the patient is conscious and respiratory secretions are not too distressing, it may be more appropriate to use a transdermal patch (Scopoderm 1.5mg over 3d.) or sublingual tablets (Kwells™). Dry mouth is a side-effect.

Terminal breathlessness: Distressing symptom for patients/carers.

Management: Support carers in attendance and explain management.

- Diamorphine or morphine: dose depends on whether the patient is being converted from oral morphine (or an alternative opioid) to diamorphine. If no previous opioid, start diamorphine 5mg/24h. s/cut. If previously on oral morphine, divide the total 24h. dose by 3 to obtain the 24h. s/cut dose of diamorphine. ↑ dose slowly as needed.
- Midazolam 5–10mg/24h. s/cut.
- If sticky secretions, try nebulized saline ± physiotherapy.

GP Notes: Syringe drivers

Although drugs can usually be administered by mouth to control the symptoms of terminal illness, occasionally that is not possible. Portable syringe drivers give a continuous subcutaneous infusion and can provide good control of symptoms with little discomfort or inconvenience to the patient. *Indications:*

- The patient is unable to take medicines by mouth owing to nausea and vomiting, dysphagia, severe weakness, or coma
- There is bowel obstruction and further surgery is inappropriate
- The patient does not want to take regular medication by mouth.

Drugs which can be used in syringe drivers

Indication	Drugs
Nausea and vomiting	Haloperidol 2.5–10mg/24h.
	Levomepromazine 5–200mg/24h. (causes sedation in 50%)
	Cyclizine 150mg/24h. (may precipitate if mixed with other drugs)
	Metoclopramide 30–100mg/24h.
	Octreotide 300–600mcgm/24h. (consultant supervision)
	Hyoscine hydrobromide 20–60mg/24h.
Respiratory secretions	Hyoscine hydrobromide 0.6–2.4mg/24h.
	Glycopyrronium 0.6–1.2mg/24h.
Restlessness and confusion	Haloperidol 5–15mg/24h.
	Levomepromazine 50–200mg/24h.
	Midazolam 20–100mg/24h. (and fitting)
Pain control	Diamorphine $\frac{1}{3}$–$\frac{1}{2}$ dose oral morphine/24h.

Mixing drugs in syringe drivers: Provided there is evidence of compatibility, drugs can be mixed in syringe drivers. Diamorphine can be mixed with:

- Cyclizine
- Hyoscine hydrobromide
- Hyoscine butylbromide
- Midazolam
- Dexamethasone
- Levomepromazine
- Haloperidol
- Metoclopramide

Common problems with syringe drivers

- *If the syringe driver runs too slowly:* Check it is switched on; check the battery; check the cannula is not blocked.
- *If the syringe driver runs too quickly:* Check the rate setting.
- *Injection site reaction:* If there is pain or inflammation, change the injection site.

🚫 Subcutaneous infusion solution should be monitored regularly both to check for precipitation (and discoloration) and to ensure the infusion is running at the correct rate.

⚠ Incorrect use of syringe drivers is a common cause of drug errors.

Chapter 5

Benefits and legal aspects of care in the community

Benefits

⚠ Information in this section is up to date at the time of going to press but benefits issues change rapidly.

Millions of pounds of benefits go unclaimed every year. This chapter is a rough guide to the benefits available to enable GPs to point their patients in the right direction. It is not intended as a comprehensive reference.

Table 5.1 Guide to agencies involved in delivering benefits to patients

Agency	Function	Website: http://www. + suffix	Telephone
Department of Work and Pensions (DWP)	Administers all benefits except: Tax credits (Inland Revenue) Statutory Sick Pay (employer) Housing benefit (local authority) Council Tax Benefit (local authority)	dwp.gov.uk	*Benefits enquiry line –* 0800 882200 *Help with form completion –* 0800 441144 *Information for employers and the self-employed –* 0845 7143143
Jobcentre Plus	Helps people of working age to find work and get any benefits they are entitled to	jobcentreplus.gov.uk	Contact local office (list available on website)
Pension Service	Provides services and support for pensioners and people looking into pensions and retirement	thepensionservice.gov.uk	Contact area office (list available on website)
Inland Revenue	Administers tax credits	hmrc.gov.uk	Tax credit enquiry line – 0845 300 3900
Disability and Carers Service	Delivers a range of benefits to disabled people and their carers	disability.gov.uk	Contact local disability benefits office (list available on DWP website)
Appeals Service	Provides an independent tribunal body for hearing appeals	appeals-service.gov.uk	N/A

🛈 0800 numbers are free; 0845 numbers are charged at local rate.

⚠ **Benefit fraud:** The DWP provides a freephone number which members of the public can telephone in confidence to give information about benefit fraud. ☎ 0800 85 44 40

Advice for patients

❶ Most benefits are payable from the date an enquiry is made, not from the date of diagnosis. Don't delay making enquiries about benefits.

Further information for patients and carers
Government information and services ⌨ www.direct.gov.uk
Citizens, Advice Bureau ⌨ www.adviceguide.org.uk
Age Concern ☎ 0800 00 99 66 ⌨ www.ageconcern.org.uk
Help the Aged ☎ 0800 800 65 65 ⌨ www.helptheaged.org.uk
Counsel and Care ☎ 0845 300 7585
⌨ www.counselandcare.org.uk

Further information for health professionals
Department of Work and Pensions (DWP) ⌨ www.dwp.gov.uk

Pensions

War pensions: For people injured whilst serving in the armed forces and their dependants (if injury caused or hastened death). Administered by the Veterans Agency, MoD. No time limit for claims. *Benefits:*

War disablement pension
- *Basic benefits:* Based on percentage disablement:
  - If <20% disabled – lump sum
  - If >20% disabled – weekly sum (pension).
- *Other benefits:* Allowances if severely disabled e.g.:
  - War pensioners mobility supplement – for walking difficulty. Holders can apply for the motability scheme and road tax exemption
  - Constant attendance allowance – for high levels of care.

Medical treatment: Some services and appliances may be paid for by the Veterans Agency (includes prescription charges, nursing home fees).

Further information
Veterans Agency ☎ 0800 169 22 77
🖳 www.veteransagency.mod.uk

Retirement pension: A state retirement pension is payable to women aged ≥60y. and men aged ≥65y., even if still working. Claim forms should be received automatically – if not, request one through the local Jobseeker Plus office. Pensions are taxable.

Basic pension: Flat rate amount – different for single people and married couples. If not enough National Insurance (NI) contributions have been paid amounts may ↓. >80y. – higher rate payable which is not dependent on NI contributions.

Increase for dependants: Paid if:
- The claimant's spouse is <60y. and earns under a set amount/does not receive certain other benefits
- The claimant has children (if claim made before April 2003).

Additional pension: State second pension (replaced SERPS). Based on NI contributions and earnings. Workers can opt out of the additional pension scheme, pay into a private or company scheme instead and pay lower NI.

Graduated pension: Some people may be entitled to a graduated pension. This is based on earnings between 1961 and 1975.

Extra pension: For a person who defers claiming retirement pension for up to 5y. Extra pension is payable when retirement pension is claimed.

🛈 If hospitalized, retirement pension is payable for 1y. at full rate. After 12mo., basic pension is ↓ but additional pension stays the same.

Other benefits for pensioners

- *Pension credit:* 📖 p.214
- *Free colour TV licence:* All pensioners >75y.
- *Winter fuel payment:* Annual payment to all pensioners >60y.
  Freephone advice service ☎ 0800 22 44 88
- *Cold weather payment:* 📖 p.216

Home Responsibilities Protection (HRP): Scheme which protects basic state pension for people who don't work or have low income and are caring for someone. 🖥 www.thepensionservice.gov.uk

Christmas Bonus: One-off payment made to people receiving a retirement pension or income support a few weeks before Christmas.

Table 5.2 Benefits for people with low income

	Eligibility	How to apply	Benefits gained
Income Support (IS)	• ≥18y. (16y. in some circumstances) and <60y. • Low income, <£8000 in savings (£16,000 if in residential care) and not in receipt of JSA • <16h. paid work/wk. (and partner <24h./wk.)	Form A1 from local Jobcentre Plus office	*Money* – depends on circumstances *Other benefits* – housing benefit, community tax benefit, health benefits and social fund payments. Children <5y. and pregnant women – free milk and vitamins. Children >5y. – free school meals and, in some areas, uniform grants *Christmas bonus* – 📖 p.213
Jobseekers Allowance (JSA)	• ≥19y. and <60y. (women) or <65y. (men) • Unemployed or working <16h./wk. • Capable of and available for work • Have a Jobseekers agreement that contracts the recipient to actively seek work	Apply by visiting local Jobcentre	*Contributions-based Jobseekers Allowance* – can claim for up to 26wk. Age-dependent fixed weekly payment *Income-based Jobseekers Allowance* – allowance dependent on circumstances. Entitles claimants to same benefits as Income Support (see above) *Hardship payments* – available to people disallowed JSA
Pension Credit	*Guarantee credit* – ≥60y. and income below the appropriate amount. Appropriate amount varies according to circumstances. Capital (excluding value of own home) >£6000 is deemed to count as income at the rate of £1/wk./£500 capital *Savings credit* – ≥65y. and income > savings credit starting point – currently >£114.05/wk. for a single person or >£174.05 if one of a couple. Depends on level of income and circumstances	Apply on form PC1 ☎ 0800 991234	*Money* – depends on circumstances *Other benefits* – if receiving guarantee credit: automatically eligible for housing benefit, community tax benefit and social fund payments

Working Tax Credit (WTC)	• Age ≥16y., working ≥16h./wk. and responsible for a child (<16y. or 16–19y. in full-time education) • Age ≥16y., working ≥16h./wk. and has a disability • Age ≥50y., working ≥16h./wk. and has started work after ≥6mo. of receiving 1 of certain benefits • Age ≥25y. and working ≥30h./wk.	Apply to Inland Revenue ☎ 0845 300 3900 🖳 www.hmrc.gov.uk	Tax credits – depends on adding together elements: • Basic element – paid to everyone entitled to WTC • Second adult element • Lone parent element • Working >30h./wk. (can combine both parents if have children) • Disability (if working >16h./wk.) • Severe disability (if working >16h./wk.) • Aged ≥50y. and in receipt of certain benefits before resuming work • Childcare – up to 70% childcare costs
Children's Tax Credit (CTC)	• Age ≥16y. and • Responsible for ≥1 child (<16y. or 16–19y. and in full-time education) • Family income <£50,000 pa	Apply to Inland Revenue ☎ 0845 300 3900 🖳 www.hmrc.gov.uk	Tax credits: • Family element – credit for any family eligible – if there is a child <1y. old in the family • Child element – credit for each individual child in the family – if the child is disabled/severely disabled
Health benefits	Automatic entitlement: • Age >60y. or <16y. (19y. if in full-time education) • Claiming IS or income-based JSA • Pregnant or within 1y. of childbirth By application: • Low income and • Savings <£8000	If automatic exemption, no need to claim. If not, claim using form HC1 available from pharmacies, GP surgeries and local Jobcentre Plus offices	Free: • Prescriptions • NHS dentistry • NHS eye tests and glasses • NHS wigs and fabric supports • Travel to hospital • Milk and vitamins for pregnant and breast-feeding women, and children <5y.

215

CHAPTER 5 **Benefits and legal aspects of care**

Table 5.2 (Contd.)

	Eligibility	How to apply	Benefits gained
Housing Benefit	Low income, living in rented housing *Exclusions* – full-time students without dependants, people in residential care or with savings >£16,000	Via local authority	Pays rent for up to 60wk, then need to reapply
Council Tax Benefit and Second Adult Rebate	• Council tax benefit – low income. Exclusions as for housing benefit • Second adult rebate – payable if someone who lives with you is aged >18y, does not pay rent or council tax and has low income • Council tax reduction – if single occupier or disabled • Disregarded occupants – certain people, including students, carers and children, are not counted in calculating the number of people living at a property	Via local authority	Council tax benefit – pays council tax Council tax reductions: • single occupier – 25% discount • all disregarded occupants – 50% • disabled – reduction to next lowest council tax band
The 6 Social Fund payments	• Crisis loan – anyone except students and people in residential care can apply • Budgeting loan – for large purchases. Must receive IS, pension credit or income-based JSA • Funeral payments – must receive low income benefit and be responsible for the funeral • Cold weather payments – average temperature <0°C for ≥7d. Must receive IS, pension credit or income-based JSA and live with a pensioner, child <5y, or disabled person • Maternity grant • Community care grant – 🔲 p.217	Cold weather payments – should be automatic All others claim via local Jobcentre Plus offices or 🔲 www.dwp.gov.uk	• Crisis loan – up to £1000 – interest-free loan repayable when crisis finished over 78wk. • Budgeting loan – as crisis loan • Funeral expenses – sum towards cost of funeral – usually does not cover full expenses • Cold weather payments – £8.50/wk.

Table 5.3 Benefits for disability and illness			
	Eligibility	How to apply	Amount
Statutory Sick Pay	• Employee age ≥16y. and <65y. • Incapable of work due to sickness or disability • Earning ≥ NI lower earnings limit • Unable to work ≥4d. and <28wk. (inc. days when would not normally work) • Those ineligible may be eligible for incapacity benefit or maternity allowance	Notify employer of illness – self-certification first 7d. (SC2, p.229); Med 3 after that time, p.229)	£68.20/wk. Some employers have more generous arrangements. Paid through normal pay mechanisms
Incapacity Benefit	• Not entitled to statutory sick pay (includes self-employed) • Unable to work (Med 3 certification until Personal Capability Assessment is applied when GP may be asked for short factual report or Med 4, pp.228–9) • < pensionable age • Sufficient NI contributions (unless aged <20y.)	Form SC1 available from GP surgeries, hospitals and local social security offices. If employed and unable to claim SSP – apply on form SSP1 supplied by employer	1–28wk. – £59.20/wk. 29–52wk. – £70.05/wk. >52weeks – £78.50/wk. Plus additions for dependants A higher rate is payable if <45y. when became unable to work or if over state retirement age
Community Care Grant	Receiving Income Support or income-based Jobseeker's Allowance and: • want to re-establish or help the applicant or a family member stay in the community • ease exceptional pressure on the applicant or a family member • to help with certain travel costs	Form SF300 from local social security offices or www.dwp.gov.uk	Minimum payment £30. No maximum amount
Disabled Facilities Grant	For work essential to help a disabled person live an independent life. Means tested	Apply via local housing department	Any reasonable application for funds is considered

Table 5.3 (Contd.)

	Eligibility	How to apply	Amount
Disability Living Allowance (DLA)[∇]	• Disability >3mo. and expected to last >6mo. more* • <65y, at time of application Mobility component: Help needed to get about outdoors • Higher rate – unable/virtually unable to walk (age >3y.) • Lower rate – help to find way in unfamiliar places (age >5y.) Care component: Help needed with personal care • Lower rate – attention/supervision needed for a significant proportion of the day or unable to prepare a cooked meal • Middle rate – attention/supervision throughout the day or repeated prolonged attention or watching over at night • Higher rate – 24h. attention/supervision day or terminal illness*	☎ 0800 882200 (0800 220674 in Northern Ireland) or Leaflet DS704 available from Post Offices or Using claim packs available at CAB and social security offices or 🖳 www.dwp.gov.uk	Mobility component: Higher rate – £43.45/wk. Lower rate – £16.50/wk. Care component: Higher rate – £62.25/wk. Middle rate – £41.65/wk. Lower rate – £16.50/wk.
Attendance Allowance (AA)[∇]	• Disability >3mo. and expected to last >6mo. more* • Aged ≥65y. • Not permanently in hospital or accommodation funded by the local authority • Needs attention/supervision – higher rate if 24h. care required/terminal illness*	☎ 0800 882200 (0800 220674 in Northern Ireland) or Leaflet DS704 available from Post Offices or 🖳 www.dwp.gov.uk	Lower rate – £41.65 Higher rate – £62.25 (for people who need day and night care or are terminally ill)

[∇] No need to receive help to apply. Not means tested.

* Terminal illness (not expected to live >6mo.) – claim under Special Rules. Claims are processed much faster and the highest care rate is automatically awarded. GP or hospital specialist fills in form DS1500 to provide clinical information to support application (fee can be claimed).

| Carer's Allowance | • Aged ≥6y. *and*
• Spends ≥35h./wk. caring for a person with a disability who is getting AA or Constant Attendance Allowance or middle or higher rate care component of DLA *and*
• Earning ≤£84.00/wk. after allowable expenses
• Not in full-time education | Complete form in leaflet DS700 available from local social security offices or
🖥 www.dwp.gov.uk | £46.95/wk.
Plus additions for dependants
(❶ No new claims for dependent children have been accepted since April 2003) |

❶

People who need someone's help to get out of the house are entitled to free prescriptions.
Severe Disablement Allowance is still paid to those who applied prior to April 2001.

Table 5.4 Mobility for disabled and elderly people ● Local public transport schemes also exist.

	Eligibility	How to apply	Benefits gained
Blue Badge Scheme	Age >2y. and ≥1 of the following: • War pensioner's mobility supplement • Higher rate of the mobility component of DLA • Motor vehicle supplied by a government health department • Registered blind • Severe disability in both upper limbs preventing turning of a steering wheel • Permanent and substantial difficulty walking	Apply through local social services department ● In most circumstances the disabled person does not have to be the driver. The badge should not be used if the disabled person is not in the car 🖵 www.dft.gov.uk	Entitles holder to park: • in specified disabled spaces • free of charge or time limit at parking meters or other places where waiting is limited • on single yellow lines for up to 3h. (no time limit in Scotland)
Motability Scheme	• Higher rate mobility component of DLA or • War pension mobility supplement ● Driver may be someone else	Contact Motability. Application guide available at 🖵 www.motability.co.uk	Registered charity. Mobility payments can be used to lease or hire-purchase a car, powered scooter or wheelchair. Grants may also be available for advance payments, adaptations or driving lessons
Road tax exemption	• Higher rate mobility component of DLA or • War pension mobility supplement or • Person nominated as someone who regularly drives for a disabled person or • Certain types of powered invalid carriages	Usually received automatically. If not and claiming DLA ☎ 0845 7123456. If claiming war pension ☎ 0800 1692277	Exemption from road tax
Seatbelt exemption	Certain medical conditions e.g. colostomy	Medical practitioner must complete exemption certificate	Exemption from wearing seatbelt

Table 5.5 Adaptations and equipment for elderly and disabled people • All purchases related to disability are VAT exempt.

	Eligibility	How to apply	Benefits received
Wheelchairs	Anyone requiring a wheelchair(s) for >3mo. Short-term loan of equipment is often available via the Red Cross	Referral by GP or specialist to wheelchair service centre. Directory service centres available at 🖳 www.wheelchairmanagers.nhs.uk	Provision of suitable wheelchair. Vouchers enable disabled patients to purchase their chairs privately
Occupational therapy (OT) assessment	All elderly or disabled people	Request needs assessment by occupational therapist via local social services department	Enables provision of equipment and adaptations necessary to maintain an independent lifestyle
Disabled Living Centres/ Disability Living Foundation	All elderly or disabled people	49 Disabled Living Centres in the UK – list available at 🖳 www.dlcc.co.uk Disabled Living Foundation ☎ 0845 130 9177 🖳 www.dlf.org.uk	Disabled Living Centres – look at and try out equipment with OTs on hand to advise Disabled Living Foundation – information on aids and adaptations
Telephone	People who have physical difficulty using the telephone or communication problems	British Telecom produce a booklet 'Communication Solutions' obtainable from ☎ 0800 800150 or 🖳 www.bt.com If difficulty using a telephone directory, register to use directory enquiries free ☎ 0800 5870195	Gadgets and services that make it easier for disabled or elderly people to use the telephone
Alarm systems	Any disabled or elderly person who is alone at times, at risk and mentally capable of using an alarm system	Arrange via local social services or housing department. Alternatively charities for the elderly have schemes (Help the Aged – Seniorlink ☎ 01255 473 999; Age Concern – Aid-Call ☎ 0800 772266)	Enables a call for help when the phone cannot be reached

Support of informal carers

In the UK there are 6 million informal carers who are vitally important to the well-being of disabled people in the community. Most are relatives or friends of the person being cared for. Many are elderly with health problems themselves. There is good evidence their health suffers as a result of caring – 52% report treatment for a stress-related illness since becoming a carer and 51% report being physically injured as a result of caring.

GPs and their primary care teams are often the 1st point of access for any help needed and 88% of carers have seen their GP in the past 12mo. Carers see the GP as the professional most able to improve their lives but few GPs have had any training about their problems and 71% carers believe their GPs are unaware of their needs.

Physical help: Record whether a patient is a carer in their notes.
- *Practical advice on nursing skills:* Ask DNs to review problems.
- *Advice on management:* Specialist nurses (e.g. respiratory nurses, cancer care nurses or Macmillan nurses etc.) provide special expertise.
- *Additional help:* Social services can provide home care. Voluntary organizations provide sitting services e.g. Crossroads schemes. Every carer has a right to ask for a full assessment of their needs by the social services.
- *Home modification:* Local authorities can arrange modifications. DNs have access to equipment needed for nursing. The Red Cross loans commodes, wheelchairs etc.
- *Respite:* Hospitals, charity organizations and local authorities provide day care (to give regular breaks each week) and respite care (for a week or more at a time).

Emotional support
- *Self-help carers' groups:* Opportunity to share experiences with people in similar situations.
- *Always ask the carer how they are when visiting,* even if they are not your patient themselves.
- *If the patient and/or carer have a religion, the clergy will often provide ongoing support.*
- *Maintain good lines of communication:* Treat the carer as a team member. Make sure you inform both carer and patient fully. Make appointments for review. Don't be short with a carer, patronising or impossible to contact.

Financial support: Many patients who have carers are entitled to Attendance Allowance or Disability Living Allowance (📖 p.218). If the patient is not expected to live >6mo. they are entitled to claim under Special Rules. This benefit is *not* means tested. Other benefits:
- *Low income* – 📖 p.214
- *Given up work to look after the patient* – may be eligible for carers allowance – 📖 p.219
- *Substantial modification to home* – council tax may be payable at lower rate (consult local council).

GMS contract

Management 9	The practice has a protocol for the identification of carers and a mechanism for the referral of carers for social services assessment	3 points

Carer support is a directed enhanced service in Scotland since April 2006

Advice for patients: Support organizations for carers

Carers UK ☎ 020 7490 8818 🖳 www.carersonline.org.uk

Princess Royal Trust for Carers ☎ 020 7480 7788
🖳 www.carers.org

Support organizations for the patient's condition (e.g. Asthma UK –
📖 p.258)

Department of Work and Pensions ☎ Benefits enquiry line
0800 882200; 0800 243355 (minicom facility); 0800 441144 (for
help with form completion) 🖳 www.dwp.gov.uk

Citizens' Advice Bureau 🖳 www.adviceguide.org.uk

Age Concern ☎ 0800 00 99 66 🖳 www.ageconcern.org.uk

Help the Aged ☎ 0800 800 65 65 🖳 www.helptheaged.org.uk

Counsel and Care ☎ 0845 300 7585
🖳 www.counselandcare.org.uk

GP Notes: Carer skills

A carer skills course is being developed for the Expert Patient
programme. Further information is available at:
🖳 www. expertpatient.nhs.uk

Occupational illness

If a patient develops an occupational disease, a doctor is obliged to notify the employer in writing with the patient's consent. The doctor does not need to make a judgment about whether the disease is, in that particular case, caused by the occupation.

Employers must then inform the Reporting of Injuries, Diseases and Dangerous Occurrences Regulations (RIDDOR) incident contact centre (☎ 0845 300 99 23 🖳 www.riddor.gov.uk). Self-employed patients must contact RIDDOR themselves.

Patients who do not give consent for the doctor to notify their employer may allow the doctor to inform the employer's occupational health department or RIDDOR directly instead.

Notifiable industrial respiratory diseases

- Barotrauma resulting in lung or other organ damage
- Tuberculosis caused by workplace exposure to sources of infection
- Legionellosis caused by workplace exposure to sources of infection
- Cancer of bronchus or lung caused by industrial exposure to carcinogens
- Primary carcinoma of the lung where there is accompanying evidence of silicosis
- Nasal or sinus cancer caused by occupational exposure to carcinogens (wood, fibreboard, nickel and leather workers)
- Pneumoconiosis
- Byssinosis in cotton or flax workers
- Mesothelioma
- Asbestosis
- Extrinsic alveolitis caused by workplace exposure to animals, birds or fungal spores
- Occupational asthma
- Poisoning by industrial agents e.g. beryllium, lead, oxides of nitrogen

🛈 This is not a complete list – for a complete list see *RIDDOR: information for doctors* available from 🖳 www.hse.gov.uk

---

Industrial injury: Injured employees should always report details of the accident to their employer and record them in the accident book as soon as possible, however trivial the injury. Employers must inform RIDDOR of:
- dangerous incidents, even if no one was hurt
- incidents where death or serious injury occurs
- incidents resulting in injury requiring >3d. absence from work
- incidents involving gas.

Industrial injuries disablement benefit: Available to employed earners for injuries resulting from accidents or certain (prescribed) illness arising as a result of employment, even if the employee was either part or wholly to blame. Industrial covers virtually all forms of work. For accidents, claims can be made at any time after the event but benefit is paid only if there are still effects of the injury after the 91st day.

GP Notes: Compensation for workers disabled by lung disease

Pneumoconiosis etc. (Workers' Compensation) Act 1979: For sufferers of certain industrial diseases caused by dust, irrespective of industry. If the patient has died, a dependant may claim. Sufferers must be unable to claim damages from the employers who caused the disease, because they have ceased trading. The sufferer or dependants must not have brought a court action or received compensation from an employer in respect of the disease.

Diseases covered:
- Diffuse mesothelioma
- Pneumoconiosis (including silicosis, asbestosis and kaolinosis) – except former coal industry workers who are covered by a separate scheme (below)
- Diffuse pleural thickening
- Primary lung cancer if accompanied by asbestosis or diffuse pleural thickening
- Byssinosis.

❶ Sufferers should normally be in receipt of disablement benefit (📖 p.226) for the disease. Dependants can claim disablement benefit posthumously but there are time limits for the claim – if time-barred, dependants can still make a claim.

Further information: ☎ 0800 279 23 22
🖥 www.jobcentreplus.gov.uk

Coal miners: Former coal industry workers suffering from pneumoconiosis, chronic bronchitis and/or COPD are covered by a separate scheme administered on behalf of the Department of Trade and Industry (☎ 0114 203 4359).

Asbestos-related disease
Government: Does NOT apply to non-employees.
- Industrial injuries disablement benefit – 📖 p.226 – next of kin can claim up to 6mo. posthumously.
- War Disablement Pensions scheme – 📖 p.212 – if exposure as a result of work in the armed forces.
- Pneumoconiosis etc. (Workers' Compensation) Act – above – if no claim can be made against the employer.

Courts
- Claims are frought with difficulty. Expert legal advice from a lawyer specializing in asbestos compensation claims is essential.
- Victims must establish their condition was caused by work and due to negligence on the part of their employers or someone else.
- Sufferers or their dependants can make claims against a previous employer, the company responsible for their exposure (e.g. exposure due to living near an asbestos factory or exposure of a spouse due to washing clothes etc.) or the company's insurer.
- Usually claims must be initiated <3y. after diagnosis of an asbestos-related disease.

Prescribed industrial disease: Disease for which benefit is paid if the applicant worked in a job for which that disease is 'prescribed' and it is likely the employment caused the disease. Claims may be made at any time with the exceptions of occupational deafness (claim <5y. after leaving employment) and occupational asthma (claim <10y. after leaving employment). The list of prescribed diseases is similar to but *not* the same as the list of notifiable diseases.

Benefits that may be payable

Disablement Benefit: If the person was a paid employee at the time of the accident or when s/he contracted the disease, *and* disability is assessed at ≥14% (exceptions: occupational deafness >20%; dust-related lung disease – no level). If a patient claims benefit for >1 industrial accident or disease, assessments may be added together and benefit awarded on the total.

Reduced Earnings Allowance: Accident occurred/disease contracted prior to 1st October 1990, disablement assessment of ≥1% *and*
• unable to work *or*
• unable to work at normal job *or*
• working less hours at normal job.

Retirement Allowance: Reduced Earnings Allowance becomes Retirement Allowance at age 60y. (woman) or 65y. (man). It is paid at 25% the rate of Reduced Earnings Allowance when a claimant stopped work.

Constant Attendance Allowance: For people so disabled they need constant care and attention and who are getting Disablement Benefit for disability assessed at 100%. 4 rates of benefit.

Exceptionally Severe Disablement Allowance: For people who get Constant Attendance Allowance at high rate and where need for attendance is likely to be permanent.

Making claims: through local Jobcentre Plus or social security office. A full list of prescribed industrial diseases is also available from these places. Some claims can be made on-line:
🖳 www.jobcentreplus. gov.uk

Further information
RIDDOR incident contact centre ☎ 0845 300 99 23
🖳 www.riddor.gov.uk
Health and Safety Executive ☎ 0870 154 55 00
🖳 www.hse.gov.uk
Jobcentre Plus 🖳 www.jobcentreplus.gov.uk
Occupational and Environmental Diseases Association
🖳 www.oeda.demon.co.uk
Trade unions

GP Notes:

❶ People who suffer from industrial diseases or have suffered disability as a result of an industrial accident are also eligible to apply for benefits available for any disabled individual – 📖 pp.218–20.

⚠ Refer all deaths, where work is thought to have contributed to death, to the coroner.

Certifying fitness to work

Own Occupation Test: Applies for the first 28wk. of their illness to those claiming:
- Statutory sick pay from their employer
- Incapacity benefit who have done a substantial amount of work in the 21wk. prior to the illness.

The doctor assesses whether the patient is fit to do their *own* job.

Personal Capability Assessment (formerly the 'All Work Test'). Assesses a patient on a variety of different mental and physical health dimensions for ability to work. Not diagnosis dependent. Applies to:
- everyone after 28wk. incapacity
- those who do not qualify for the Own Occupation Test from the start of their incapacity.

Claimants are sent form IB50 to complete themselves and are asked to obtain form Med4 from their GP. If the Department of Work and Pensions (DWP) is not happy to continue paying their benefit on the basis of these reports, the applicant is called for a medical examination. Conditions relevant to respiratory disease which exempt patients from further examination include:
- Receipt of highest rate care component of Disability Living Allowance (DLA), Constant Attendance Allowance or >80% disabled for other benefit purposes
- Terminal illness
- Progressive immune deficiency (including AIDS)
- Severe progressive cardio-respiratory disease which persistently limits exercise tolerance.

Private certificates: Some employers request private certificates in the 1st week of sickness absence. They should request it in writing. If the GP chooses to provide the service, (s)he may charge both for a private consultation and the provision of a private certificate. The company should accept full responsibility for all fees incurred by the patient.

Permitted work: Incapacity benefits do allow very limited work – therapeutic work (must be done as part of a treatment programme and in an institution which provides sheltered work for people with disabilities); voluntary work; local authority councillor; disability expert on an appeal tribunal or member of the Disability Living Allowance advisory board (not >1d./wk.).

Disability Discrimination Act 1995: In some circumstances requires employers to make reasonable adjustments for an employee with a long-term disability. Advise patients to seek specialist advice.

Disability Employment Advisors: Provided by the Employment Service to assist disabled patients to get back to work. Contacted by:
- Writing a comment to the effect that intervention would be helpful in the comments box on form Med3 *or*
- Writing to the local Jobcentre Plus (with the patient's permission).

Table 5.6 Forms for certifying incapacity to work

Form	Use
SC1	Self-certification form for people not eligible to claim statutory sick pay who wish to claim incapacity benefit. Certifies first 7d. of illness. Available from local Jobcentre Plus offices and GP surgery.
SC2	As SC1 but for people who can claim statutory sick pay. Available from employer, local Jobcentre Plus offices and GP surgery.
Med 3	Filled in by GP or hospital doctor who knows the patient for periods of incapacity to work likely to be >7d. If return within 14d. is forecast give fixed date of return ('closed certificate'). If longer, specify a period of time (e.g. 2mo.) ('open certificate'). Before the patient returns to work reassess and give further certificate with fixed date of return. Only one Med3 can be issued per patient per period of sickness. If mislaid, reissue and mark 'duplicate'.
Med 4	See Personal Capability Assessment (opposite). Only completed once for any period of incapacity from work.
Med 5	Can be used if: • A doctor has not seen the patient but on the basis of a recent (<1mo.) written report from another doctor is satisfied that the patient should not work – the certificate should not cover a forward period of >1mo. • The patient returned to work without receiving a closed certificate (see Med3 above) • >1d. since the patient was seen (so Med3 or Med4 cannot be issued) but it is clear the disability is ongoing.
Med 6	Used when it is felt that putting a diagnosis on a Med3/Med4 would be harmful either directly to a patient or through their employer knowing their diagnosis. A vague diagnosis is put on the form and a Med6 completed which requests the Department of Works and Pensions (DWP) to send a form to obtain more precise details.
RM 7	Sent directly to the DWP to request review of the patient by them sooner than would usually be undertaken.

GP Notes: Useful information

Department of Work and Pensions *Medical Evidence for Statutory Sick Pay, Statutory Maternity Pay and Social Security Incapacity Benefit Purposes: a guide for registered medical practitioners.* IB204. April 2000
🖥 www.dwp.gov.uk/medical/medicalib204/index.asp
Disability Discrimination Act 🖥 www.disability.gov.uk

Fitness to drive

> ⚠ Driving licence holders (or applicants) have a legal duty to inform the DVLA of any disability likely to cause danger to the public if they were to drive.

Driving licence types

- **Group 1:** Ordinary licence for driving a car/motorcycle. Old licences expire at 70th birthday and then must be renewed 3-yearly. Applicants are asked to confirm they have no medical disability. If so, no medical examination is necessary. New photocard licences are automatically renewed 10-yearly until age 70y. Minimum age 17y. (16y. if disabled).
- **Group 2:** Enable holders to drive lorries and buses. Min. age 21y. Initially valid until 45th birthday then renewable every 5y. until 65th birthday. >65y. renewable annually. Medical examination is needed to renew group 2 licences. Applicants must bring form D4 (available from post offices) with them. Examinations take ~½ h. A fee may be charged by the GP.

Determining fitness to drive: Patients with any disorder which may cause danger to others if they drove should be advised not to drive and contact the DVLA. The DVLA gives advice on when they can restart.

Specific guidance regarding respiratory conditions: Table 5.7

GP Notes: What should I do if a patient continues to drive despite advice to stop?

If the patient does not understand the advice to stop driving: inform the DVLA.

If the patient does understand the advice to stop driving:
- Explain your legal duty to breach confidentiality and inform the DVLA if they do not stop driving.
- If the patient still refuses to stop driving, offer a second medical opinion – on the understanding they stop driving in the interim.
- If the patient still continues driving, consider action such as recruiting next-of-kin to the cause – but beware of breach of confidentiality.
- If all else fails, write to the patient to inform him/her of your intention to inform the DVLA.
- If the patient continues to drive, inform the DVLA and write to the patient to confirm a disclosure has been made.

🛈 Always consider contacting your medical defence body for advice.

Table 5.7 DVLA guidance about fitness to drive for patients with respiratory problems

Condition	Group 1 licence restrictions	Group 2 licence restrictions
Sleep disorders (causing excessive daytime or awake-time sleepiness)	Inform DVLA. Stop driving until symptoms are controlled – must be confirmed by a doctor.	Inform DVLA. Stop driving until symptoms are controlled, with ongoing compliance with treatment – must be confirmed by a consultant. When restored, subject to regular licensing review – usually annually.
Cough syncope	Inform DVLA. Stop driving until liability to attacks has been successfully controlled – must be confirmed by a doctor.	Inform DVLA Stop driving. If chronic respiratory condition (including smoking) – restored if free from syncope/pre-syncope for 5y. If asystole due to coughing, licence may be restored after pacemaker fitted.
Respiratory disorders e.g. asthma, COPD	No need to notify DVLA unless associated with disabling giddiness, fainting or loss of consciousness.	As for group 1.
Carcinoma of the lung	No need to notify DVLA unless cerebral secondaries. If cerebral secondaries, stop driving and notify DVLA.	Inform DVLA. Non-small-cell lung cancer classified as T1N0M0 – DVLA considers each case on an individual basis. All other lung cancer – stop driving until 2y. after definitive treatment. Driving may resume providing treatment is satisfactory and there is no brain scan evidence of intracranial metastases.

Further information

DVLA *At a glance guide to the current medical standards of fitness to drive for medical practitioners* available from 🖥 www.dvla.gov.uk

Medical advisers from the DVLA can advise on difficult issues – contact: Drivers Medical Unit, DVLA, Swansea SA99 1TU or ☎ 01792 761119

Fitness to fly

Passengers are required to tell the airline at the time of booking about any conditions that might compromise their fitness to fly. The airline's medical officer must then decide whether to carry them or not. Respiratory conditions are the 3rd most common cause of in-flight emergency.

Hazards of flying

- Cabin pressure – oxygen levels are lower than at ground level and gas in body cavities expands 30% in flight
- Inactivity and dehydration
- Disruption of routine
- Alcohol consumption
- Stress and excitement

Respiratory illnesses which prevent flying

- *Pneumothorax:* Should not fly for 6wk. after complete resolution of pneumothorax. At ↑ risk of recurrence due to flying for up to 1y.
- *Acute infectious disease*
- *Infectious TB*
- *SARS:* Contacts of probable or confirmed cases

Patients who may need further assessment prior to flying

- Patients with oxygen saturations of <95% in air
- Patients with severe airways disease e.g. COPD, asthma, fibrosing alveolitis, cystic fibrosis
- Patients hospitalized for a respiratory disease in the preceding 6wk.
- Patients with a history of respiratory problems in the past on flying
- Patients with neuromuscular disease
- Patients with significant kyphosis/scoliosis causing a ventilatory deficit
- Patients with other conditions worsened by hypoxaemia e.g. coronary/cerebro-vascular disease, heart failure

❶ As a rule of thumb, patients able to walk 50m without distress off oxygen are fit to fly. If in doubt, seek advice from the consultant in charge of the patient's care.

Specific conditions

- *Asthma:* If stable, is not usually a problem, as long as patients take their inhlaers with them. Battery operated nebulizers can be used during flights but not during take off/landing – inform the airline in advance.
- *COPD:* Patients able to walk >50m without distress off oxygen are fit to fly. Even if patients are unable to walk >50m without distress off oxygen, they may be able to fly with supplementary oxygen. Get specialist advice. Oxygen must be booked in advance through the airline and there is usually an additional charge.
- *Obstructive sleep apnoea:* Avoid alcohol before and during flight. If significant desaturation during sleep, consider using CPAP on overnight flights – discuss with the airline.

Further information

British Thoracic Society Managing patients with respiratory disease planning air travel *Thorax* (2002) **57**: 289–304.

GP Notes: Travel

Long-haul flights and DVT/PE: Advise *all* patients to:
- Drink plenty of non-alcoholic fluids
- Keep their legs moving whilst sitting, or walk up and down the aisle.

Graduated compression hosiery is available for purchase OTC and does ↓ risk of DVT, but is unnecessary for most people. Consider recommending for patients who:
- Are taking the COC pill or HRT
- Have a chronic illness e.g. inflammatory bowel disease
- Have recently (<72h.) had minor surgery
- Have extensive varicose veins
- Have polycythaemia *or*
- Are relatively immobile (e.g. elderly, obese, disabled).

Consider pre-flight aspirin (300mg) and graduated compression stockings if:
- Family history of venous thromboembolism
- Pregnant or in the early postnatal period
- Leg trauma or paralysis

Anticoagulation
- Those with a history of DVT/PE during flight or thrombophilia (if not already anticoagulated) need heparin cover – refer for specialist advice.
- Consider anticoagulation with low-molecular-weight heparin (if not already anticoagulated) if <6wk. after major surgery, previous stroke or current malignancy – take specialist advice.

Altitude: Patients travelling to high altitude destinations may have difficulty with their breathing, particularly if underlying lung disease. Warn patients to seek medical advice promptly if they have any breathing problems and discourage patients with significant lung disease or restriction of lung capacity from travelling to high altitude destinations.

Insurance: Any person travelling abroad should take out comprehensive travel insurance including medical and repatriation expenses. Inform insurance companies of any pre-existing disease prior to travel. If illness occurs whilst abroad, inform the insurer as soon as possible – most have helplines for such eventualities.

Medication: Always carry essential medication and medication which might be needed during flight in hand luggage.

❶ For patients or doctors travelling abroad with schedule 2 or 3 drugs, an export licence may be required. Further details can be obtained from the Home Office (☎ 020 7273 3806). Patient applications must be accompanied by a doctor's letter giving details of:
- Patient's name, current address and dates of travel
- Quantities, strength and form of drugs to be carried.

⚠ For clearance to import a drug into the country of destination, it is advisable to contact the Embassy or High Commission of that country prior to departure.

233

Fitness to perform other activities

Fitness to perform sporting activities: GPs are commonly asked to certify fitness to perform sports. Normally the patient will come with a medical form. If there is a form, request to see it before the medical. If there is no form and you are unsure what to check, telephone the sport's governing body or the event organizer. A fee is payable by the patient.

Many gyms and sports clubs also ask older patients and patients with pre-existing conditions or disabilities to check with their GP before they will sign them on. Assuming that a suitable regime is undertaken most people can participate in some form of sporting activity. Consider the patient's baseline fitness, check BP and medications and recommend a gradual introduction to any new forms of exercise.

Diving: Respiratory fitness is essential for diving. Before diving, prospective divers must obtain a medical certificate stating they are fit.

Diving medicals should include
- Assessment of respiratory history – current and previous respiratory problems (including childhood problems)
- Respiratory examination including assessment of lung function (PEFR ± spirometry)
- CXR – if professional diver or diving instructor, previous significant respiratory illness, current symptoms or abnormal examination.

Contraindications to diving include
- Lung bullae or cysts
- COPD
- Active TB
- Cystic fibrosis
- Fibrotic lung disease.

Specific circumstances
- Pneumothorax – history of spontaneous pneumothorax is a contraindication. Traumatic pneumothorax is not if completely resolved.
- Asthma – may dive if free of asthma symptoms, normal spirometry and negative exercise test (<15% fall in PEFR after exercise).
- Sarcoid – contraindicated if active. Allowed after normal CXR.

Pre-employment certification: It is becoming increasingly common for GPs to be asked about the 'medical' suitability of candidates to perform a job. This is not part of the GP's terms of service and therefore a GP can refuse to give an opinion. In all cases where an opinion is given, a fee can be claimed. Common examples are:
- Ofsted forms for childminders
- Care home staff – proof of 'physical and mental fitness'
- Food handlers – certificates of fitness.

Further information
British Thoracic Society Guidelines on respiratory aspects of fitness for diving *Thorax* (2003) **58**: 3–13 ⬚ www.brit-thoracic.org.uk

Advance directives/Living wills: Statements in which a person makes a decision about medical treatment in case he or she becomes incapable of making that decision later.
- Respect any refusal of treatment given when the patient was competent, provided the decision is clearly applicable to present circumstances and was not made under duress
- The BMA recommends doctors do *not* withhold 'basic care' (e.g. symptom control) even if the patient has specified 'no treatment'
- Where an advance directive is not available, take patient's known wishes into consideration.

GP Notes: Fitness to perform certificates

⚠ Remember – signing a form may result in legal action against you should the patient NOT be fit to undertake an activity.

Where possible include a caveat e.g. 'Based on information available in the medical notes the patient appears to be fit to…, although it is impossible to guarantee this.'

If unsure, consult your local LMC or medical defence organization for advice.

235

Chapter 6

The General Medical Services contract and respiratory problems

The General Medical Services (GMS) contract

Although there may be some differences in process in each of the four countries of the UK, the principles of the GMS contract apply to all. A total sum for GMS services is given to each primary care organization (PCO) as part of a bigger unified budget allocation. PCOs are responsible for managing the GMS budget locally.

The contract: Made between an individual practice and a PCO. All the partners of the practice, at least one of whom must be a GP, have to sign the contract. It includes:
- National terms applicable to all practices (the 'practice contract')
- Which services will be provided by that practice i.e.
  - essential
  - additional – if not opted out
  - out-of-hours – if not opted out
  - enhanced – if opted in
- Level of quality of essential and additional services that the practice 'aspires' to
- Support arrangements e.g. IT, premises
- Total financial resources i.e. global sum + quality achievement payments + enhanced services payments + premises + IT + dispensing.

Essential services: All practices must undertake these services.
Include:
- ***Day-to-day medical care of the practice population:*** health promotion, management of minor and self-limiting illness and referral to secondary care services and other agencies as appropriate
- ***General management of patients who are terminally ill***
- ***Chronic disease management.***

Additional services: Services the practice will usually undertake but may 'opt out' of. If the practice opts out, the PCO takes responsibility for providing the service instead. The practice then receives a ↓ global sum payment.

Enhanced services: Commissioned by the PCO and paid for *in addition* to the global sum payment. 3 types:
- ***Directed enhanced services:*** services under national direction with national specifications and benchmark pricing which all PCOs must commission to cover their relevant population
- ***National enhanced services:*** services with national minimum standards and benchmark pricing but not directed (i.e. PCOs do not have to provide these services)
- ***Services developed locally*** to meet local needs (local enhanced services) e.g. enhanced care of the homeless.

Table 6.1 Payment under the GMS contract

Payment	Explanation
The global sum	Major part of the money paid to practices. Paid monthly and intended to cover practice running costs. Includes provision for: • Delivery of essential services and additional/ out-of-hours services if not opted out • Staff costs • Career development • Locum reimbursement (e.g. for appraisal, career development and protected time).
Aspiration payments	Advance payments to allow practices to develop services to achieve higher quality standards. Practices agree their aspirations for quality points the following year with their PCO. Aspiration payments are made monthly alongside global sum payments and amount to roughly 60% of the points achieved the previous year (for 2005/6 this was ≈ 2004/5 points achieved × £ 124.60/point × 60% × adjustment for list size and composition).
Achievement payments	Payments made for the practice's achieved number of points in the Quality and Outcomes Framework (📖 p.240) as measured at the start of the following year. Aspiration payments already received are deducted from the total i.e. payment for actual points less aspiration pay.
Payment for 'extra' services	Paid to practices that provide enhanced services, national enhanced services and/or local enhanced services to meet local needs.
Minimum practice income guarantee (MPIG)	Protects those practices that lost out under the redistribution effect of the new resource allocation formula. Calculated from the difference between the global sum allocation (GSA) under the new GMS contract and the global sum equivalent (GSE) – the amount the practice would have earned for providing the same service under the old GMS contract ('The Red Book'). If GSA < GSE a correction factor (CF) will be applied as long as necessary so that GSA + CF = GSE.
Other payments	Payments for premises, IT and dispensing (dispensing practices only).

239

❗ The Carr-Hill allocation formula is a GMS resource allocation formula for allocating funds for the global sum and quality payments. The formula takes the practice population and then makes a series of adjustments based on the profile of the local community, taking account of determinants of relative practice workload and costs.

The Quality and Outcomes Framework

The Quality and Outcomes Framework (QOF) was developed specifically for the new GMS contract. Financial incentives are used to encourage high quality care.

The domains: The GMS Quality Framework is divided into 4 domains:

- Clinical
- Organizational
- Additional services
- Patient experience

See Table 6.2

Indicators: Every domain has a set of 'indicators' which relate to quality standards or guidelines that can be achieved within that domain. The indicators were developed by an expert group based on the best available evidence at the time and will be updated regularly. All data should be obtainable from practice clinical systems and Read codes have been developed to make this easier. Indicators are split into 3 types:

- *Structure* e.g. is a disease register in place?
- *Process:* e.g. is a particular measure being recorded? Is action being taken where appropriate?
- *Outcome:* e.g. how well is the condition being controlled?

Quality points: All achievement against quality indicators converts to points. Each point has a monetary value.

- *Yes/no indicators:* All points are allocated if the result is +ve and none if −ve.
- *Range of attainment:* For most of the clinical indicators it is not possible to attain 100% results (even if allowed exceptions are applied) so a range of satisfactory attainment is specified. Points are allocated in a linear fashion based on comparison with attainment against a maximum standard e.g. if the maximum % for an indicator is 90%, the minimum 40% and the practice achieves 65%, the practice will receive 25/50 (i.e. 1/2) of the available points.

Reporting on quality: Every year each practice must complete a standard return form recording level of achievement and the evidence for that. In addition there is an annual quality review visit by the PCO. Based on these, the PCO confirms level of achievement funding attained and discusses points the practice will 'aspire' to the following year (📖 p.239). The process is confirmed in writing by the PCO and signed off by the practice. The Commission for Healthcare Audit and Inspection (or equivalents in Scotland/NI) checks PCO-wide quality.

The Quality Framework and the Personal Medical Services (PMS) contract: Mechanisms for quality delivery and the QOF are broadly comparable for GMS and PMS practices. PMS practices can apply for aspiration payments and achievement payments in the same way as GMS practices. However, in order to reflect the local nature of the contracts, standards PMS practices are working to do not have to be the same as those contained in the national QOF. Nevertheless, all standards must be: rigorous; evidence based; monitored fairly; assessed against criteria agreed between PCOs and providers; and paid at appropriate and equitable rates.

Table 6.2 Calculation of points for Quality Framework payments		
Components of total points score	**Points**	**Way in which points are calculated**
Clinical indicators	655	Achieving pre-set standards in management of: CHD, Heart failure, Atrial fibrillation, Stroke and TIA, Hypertension, Hypothyroidism, Chronic kidney disease, DM, Obesity, Smoking, Learning disability, Mental health, Depression, Dementia, COPD, Asthma, Epilepsy, Cancer, Palliative care
Organizational	181	Achieving pre-set standards in: Records and information about patients, Information for patients, Education and training, Medicines management, Practice management.
Additional services	36	Achieving pre-set standards in: Cervical screening, Child health surveillance, Maternity services, Contraceptive services.
Patient experience	108	Achieving pre-set standards in: Patient survey*, Consultation length.
Holistic care	20	Reflects range of achievement across clinical indicators – calculated by ranking clinical indicators in terms of proportion of points gained (1–10). Proportion of the points gained by the 3rd lowest indicator (i.e. indicator ranked 7) is the proportion of the holistic care points obtained.
Total possible	**1000**	

In 2005/6 the average value of 1 point = £124.60.
* Improving Patient Questionnaire (IPQ – charge payable) – www.cfep.co.uk or General Practice Assessment Questionnaire (GPAQ) – www.gpaq.info

Further information

DoH The GMS Contract www.dh.gov.uk
BMA The Blue book and supporting documents www.bma.org.uk
NHS Employers www.nhsemployers.org/primary/index

241

COPD indicators

Maximizing points: In 2006/7, 33 points out a total of 1000 are available for COPD quality indicators.

Disease register: A register of patients who require follow up is a prerequisite for structured COPD care. COPD Indicator 1 requires the practice to 'produce a register of patients with COPD' and report the number of patients on its COPD register as a proportion of total list size.

❶ The PCO may compare reported and expected prevalence – know your inclusion and exclusion criteria and be able to justify them.

Diagnosis: COPD is diagnosed if:
- the patient has an FEV_1 of <70% of predicted normal
- *and* has an FEV_1/FVC ratio of <70%
- *and* there is a <15% response to a reversibility test.

For the quality and outcomes framework, the FEV_1 is set at 70% although other major guidelines (e.g. British Thoracic Society) state 80%. This is because many of the patients with FEV_1 <80% but >70% will have minimal symptoms. The use of the 70% cut off enables GPs to concentrate on patients with symptomatic COPD. The quality and outcomes framework requires spirometry to be used for diagnosis of all COPD patients (COPD indicator 9).

❶ Patients with reversible airways obstruction should be included in the asthma disease register. No patient should be on both the asthma and COPD disease registers.

Influenza vaccination: All patients with a history of COPD should be offered annual influenza vaccination in the autumn/winter months. Report the percentage of patients on the COPD register who have an influenza vaccination recorded for the preceding winter (COPD indicator 8).

Regular review: COPD indicators 10 and 11 require practices to review patients with COPD every 15mo. Remember to ask about smoking status (📖 p.244).

Spirometry: There is a gradual deterioration in lung function in patients with COPD. This deterioration accelerates with time. Interventions can improve quality of life in patients with severe COPD such as:
- Pulmonary rehabilitation *and/or*
- Continuous oxygen therapy

It is important to monitor respiratory function to identify patients with increasing severity of disease (FEV_1 <50% predicted or disabling symptoms) who might benefit from referral. Measure FEV_1 at least every 15mo. (COPD indicator 10).

Inhaler technique: Inhaled therapies can improve the quality of life in some patients with COPD. There is also evidence that patients require training in how to use their inhalers which should be regularly reinforced, and that poor technique is often a reason for treatment failure. The frequency of training is unclear but has been set for the purpose of the quality and outcome framework as every 15mo. (COPD indicator 11).

Table 6.3 COPD indicators

Indicator	Description	Points	Payment stages
COPD 1	The practice can produce a register of patients with COPD	3 points	
COPD 9	% of all patients with COPD in whom diagnosis has been confirmed by spirometry including reversibility testing	10 points	40–80%
COPD 8	% of COPD patients who have had influenza vaccine in the preceding 1st September – 31st March	up to 6 points	40–85%
COPD 10	% of COPD patients with a record of FEV1 in the previous 15mo.	up to 7 points	40–70%
COPD 11	% of patients with COPD receiving inhaled treatment in whom there is a record that inhaler technique has been checked in the previous 15mo.	up to 7 points	40–90%

⚠ Patients should not be on the asthma AND COPD register. If the patient was previously on the asthma register but now has COPD, code as inactive on asthma register.

Box 6.1 Exception reporting

In some circumstances the targets of the quality and outcomes framework are either not achievable through no fault of the practice, or not appropriate (e.g. if the patient is terminally ill). Under these circumstances the practice can report exceptions. Where there has been exception reporting, exceptions are subtracted from the number on the register in order to calculate the percentage. *Valid exceptions:*

- Patients who refuse to attend review who have been invited ≥3x in the preceding 12mo. (there must be a record of this)
- Patients for whom it would not be appropriate to review the disease due to particular circumstances e.g. terminal illness, extreme frailty
- Patients newly diagnosed within the practice or who have recently registered with the practice, who should have measurements made in <3mo. and delivery of clinical standards (e.g. BP or cholesterol measurement within target levels) in <9mo.
- Patients on maximum tolerated doses of medication whose levels remain sub-optimal
- Patients for whom prescribing a medication is not clinically appropriate e.g. due to allergy, another contraindication or adverse reaction
- Where a patient has not tolerated medication
- Where a patient does not agree to investigation or treatment (informed dissent), and this has been recorded in their medical records
- Where the patient has a supervening condition which makes treatment of their condition inappropriate e.g. cholesterol reduction where the patient has liver disease
- Where an investigative service or secondary care service is unavailable.

Asthma and smoking indicators

Maximizing points: In 2006/7, 45 points out a total of 1000 are available for asthma quality indicators. A further 79 points are available for recording smoking status.

Asthma:

Disease register: Proactive structured review as opposed to opportunistic/unscheduled review is associated with ↓ exacerbation rates and days lost from normal activity. A register of patients who require follow up is a prerequisite for structured asthma care. Asthma indicator 1 requires the practice to 'produce a register of patients with asthma'. Patients with quiescent asthma not requiring medication over the previous 12mo. should be excluded. The practice reports the number of patients on its asthma register as a proportion of total list size.

ⓘ The PCO may compare reported and expected prevalence – know your inclusion and exclusion criteria and be able to justify them.

Diagnosis: All diagnoses of asthma should be confirmed by demonstrating PEFR variability through serial PEFR monitoring or response to bronchodilators as measured using spirometry (Asthma indicator 8). A pragmatic age of 8y. has been specified as children younger than this may not be able to use a peak flow meter or spirometer effectively.

Smoking status of young asthma sufferers: Many people start to smoke at an early age. Smoking may ↑ the risk of persisting asthma and is associated with poor asthma control. Ask about smoking at annual review in the 14–19y. age group (Asthma indicator 3).

Regular review: Asthma indicator 6 requires practices to review patients with asthma every 15mo. The format of the review is not specified but it is suggested that reviews should include:
- Assessment of symptoms (e.g. with the RCP 3 questions – 📖 p.111)
- Measurement of PEFR
- Assessment of inhaler technique
- Consideration of provision of a personalized asthma plan.

Exception reporting: 📖 p.243

Smoking: Smoking cessation is the single most effective – and cost-effective – intervention to ↓ risk of development and progression of COPD. In asthmatics smoking is associated with poor control.
- Record whether/ how much patients are smoking (Smoking 1). If the patient has never smoked, only record smoking status once – otherwise for asthmatics and patients with COPD, record smoking status at each annual review (every 15mo.).
- Where patients have been identified as smokers, offer smoking cessation advice and/or referral to the local smoke-stop service (Smoking 2). Report the percentage of current smokers offered smoking cessation advice.

Table 6.4 Asthma indicators

Indicator	Description	Points	Payment stages
Asthma 1	The practice can produce a register of patients with asthma, excluding patients with asthma who have been prescribed no asthma-related drugs in the last 12mo.	4 points	
Asthma 8	% of patients aged ≥8y. diagnosed as having asthma from 1.4.2006 with measures of variability or reversibility	up to 15 points	40–80%
Asthma 3	% of patients with asthma aged 14–19y. in whom there is a record of smoking status in the previous 15mo.	up to 6 points	40–80%
Asthma 6	% of patients with asthma who have had an asthma review in the last 15mo.	up to 20 points	40–70%

⚠ Patients should not be on the asthma and COPD register.

Table 6.5 Smoking indicators

Indicator	Description	Points	Payment stages
Smoking 1	% of patients with any/combination of coronary heart disease, stroke or TIA, hypertension, diabetes, COPD or asthma whose notes record smoking status in the previous 15mo. Except those who have never smoked where smoking status need only be recorded once since diagnosis	up to 33 points	40–90%
Smoking 2	% of patients with any/combination of the conditions listed in 'smoking 1' who smoke whose notes contain a record that smoking cessation advice or referral to a specialist service, where available, has been offered within the previous 15mo.	up to 35 points	40–90%
Records 22	% of patients aged >15y. whose notes record smoking status in the past 27mo., except those who have never smoked where smoking status need be recorded only once.	up to 11 points	40–90%
Information 5	The practice supports smokers in stopping smoking by a strategy which includes providing literature and offering appropriate therapy.	2 points	

GP Notes:

Verification of figures supplied: PCOs may verify figures provided by inspecting computer outputs used to generate the figures; inspecting a sample of records of asthma patients; or inspecting a sample of records of patients claimed by the practice to have had a particular check e.g. spirometry or PEFR measurement, for objective evidence of that claim.

Additional and enhanced services

Vaccination as an additional service: 2 *additional service* payments are available for vaccinating patients registered as either permanent residents or temporary residents within the practice area:

- *Childhood vaccinations and immunizations:* includes all necessary childhood vaccinations and immunizations – Table 6.6
- *Vaccinations and immunizations:* includes all necessary vaccinations and immunizations (except the influenza and pneumococcal immunization directed enhanced services, childhood vaccinations and immunizations and certain travel vaccines that can be charged for privately) provided by the NHS.

In all cases the practice must:

- Provide enough information to enable informed choice about whether to have a vaccination
- Record in the patient's notes any refusal to routine vaccination
- Record in the patient's notes any contraindications to administration
- Where the offer of vaccination is accepted, record the patient's consent to the vaccination or the name of the person who gave consent and relationship to the patient
- Where the offer of vaccination is accepted, administer the vaccination and record the date of administration in the patient's notes together with the title (including manufacturer), batch number and expiry date
- Where 2 vaccines are administered in close succession, record route of administration and injection site of each vaccine in the patient notes
- Record in the patient's notes any adverse reactions to the vaccination
- Ensure all staff involved in administering vaccines are trained in the recognition and initial treatment of anaphylaxis.

Opting out of giving vaccinations:

- Routine Childhood vaccinations – 1% ↓ in global sum
- Other vaccinations – 2% ↓ in global sum

Childhood vaccination as a directed enhanced service: Requires practices to:

- Develop and maintain a register of registered children aged ≤ 5y.
- Provide information to parents about the vaccination programme and record that advice has been given in the child's GP notes.
- Record any refusal of vaccination in the child's notes
- Perform the immunizations and record it has been given in the child's notes
- Provide all necessary training for staff in order for them to advise on and administer the vaccinations
- Have resuscitation equipment on site in case of anaphylactic shock
- Audit the process – including monitoring of immunization rates in the under 2's; booster rates for the under 5's; and, changes in these rates within the year together with possible reasons for those changes.

Payment: Practices must report all immunizations given to their local PCO. Arrangements for doing this vary according to locality.

Table 6.6 UK schedule of childhood immunization		
Disease (vaccine)	**Age**	**Comment**
Tuberculosis (BCG)	High risk neonates	1 injection
Diphtheria/Tetanus/Pertussis/ Haemophilus influenzae type b/ Inactivated Polio (DTaP/IPV/Hib)	2, 3 and 4mo.	Primary course (3 doses, a month between each dose)
Pneumococcal vaccine	2, 4 and 13mo.	Primary course
Meningococcus type C (men C)	3, 4 and 12mo.	Primary course
Haemophilus influenzae type b (Hib)	12mo.	Booster dose
Measles/Mumps/Rubella (MMR)	13mo.	1st dose, 1 injection
Diphtheria/Tetanus/Acellular pertussis /inactivated Polio (DTP/IPV)	3y.4mo.-5y. (3y. after completion of the p course)	Booster dose 1 injection
Measles/Mumps/Rubella (MMR)	3y.4mo.-5y.	2nd dose, 1 injection
Tetanus/low dose diphtheria (Td/IPV)/inactivated Polio	13–18y.	Booster dose 1 injection

There are 2 payments available for childhood immunization – one for children aged 2y. and another for children aged 5y. These are paid when children complete their vaccinations.

For children aged 2 this includes:
- Group 1 – Pentavalent vaccine (diptheria, tetanus, poliomyelitis, pertussis and Hib) (50% of target payment)
- Group 2 – MMR (25% of target payment)
- Group 3 – Meningitis C (25% of target payment)

For children aged 5 this includes: A single booster dose of diptheria, tetanus, polio and pertussis.

Within each of these 2 payments, there are 2 levels of payment which depend on the % of eligible children who complete their vaccinations. The lower payment is achieved when ≥70% of eligible children have been vaccinated; the higher figure when this proportion is ≥90%.

Payments, adjusted further for the proportion of vaccinations carried out in NHS general practice or elsewhere (such as in private clinics), are made quarterly if, on the first day of the quarter, the proportion of vaccinated eligible patients on the practice list on the day is 70% or more.

🄳 Exception reporting/informed dissent *does not* apply.

Influenza and pneumococcal immunizations for at risk groups as a directed enhanced service: This directed enhanced service aims to provide influenza and pneumococcal vaccination for the elderly and other 'at-risk' groups – including those taking immunosuppressant drugs for arthritis. Practices DO NOT have preferred provider status for this service.

Target group for influenza vaccination: 📖 p.149

Target group for pneumococcal vaccination: 📖 p.155

Qualifications to provide the service:
- Practices are expected to use a call-recall system identifying those 'at-risk' through existing registers compiled for use within the quality and outcomes framework.
- Practices not participating in the quality and outcomes framework must compile a register to qualify to provide this enhanced service.

Targets:
- No target has been set for the proportion of 'at-risk' patients given influenza or pneumococcal vaccination.
- Additional payments are available through the quality and outcomes framework for vaccinating high proportions of 'at-risk' patients against influenza – but most of these targets do not currently apply to children <16y.

Anti-coagulation monitoring as a national enhanced service: This service aims to provide an anti-coagulation monitoring scheme in the community for patients started on therapy in secondary care.

Practices must:

- Develop a register of anticoagulated patients – this must include name, date of birth, indication for and length of treatment and target INR.
- Provide a call-recall system
- Educate newly diagnosed patients and provide ongoing information for established patients including provision of a patient-held booklet
- Create an individual management plan for each patient on the register
- Refer promptly to other services and relevant support agencies using local guidelines where they exist
- Review the patient's health at diagnosis and at least annually thereafter including checks for potential complications.
- Keep records of the service provided including all information relating to significant events e.g. hospital admission, death and ensure these records are included in the GP record.
- Provide ongoing training to staff involved
- Review the scheme annually including internal and external quality assurance for any computer-aided decision making equipment or near-patient testing equipment used and audit of care of patients including untoward incidents.

It is a condition of participation in the scheme that practitioners will give notification within 72h. of the information becoming available to the practitioner to the PCO clinical governance lead of all emergency admissions or deaths of any patients covered by this service, where such an admission or death is or may be due to usage of the drug(s) in question or attributable to the relevant underlying medical condition.

Funding available: Fees vary according to whether the blood is taken in the practice or not, the sample is tested in the practice or not and the dose is monitored by the practice or not. There are 4 levels of payment. In addition a fee per home visit for testing is payable.

Chapter 7

Useful information and contacts

Useful information and contacts for GPs

General information

British Thoracic Society 🖳 www.brit-thoracic.org.uk

British Lung Foundation ☎ 08458 50 50 20 🖳 www.lunguk.org

Chapman *et al. Oxford Handbook of Respiratory Medicine* (2005) Oxford University Press ISBN: 0198520775

DIPEx patient experience database 🖳 www.dipex.org

NICE Referral guidelines for suspected cancer – quick reference guide (2005) 🖳 www.nice.org.uk

National Electronic Library for Health 🖳 www.nelh.nhs.uk

Allergy/anaphylaxis

British Society for Allergy and Clinical Immunology (BSACI) 🖳 www.bsaci.org

Resuscitation Council UK Emergency medical treatment of anaphylactic reactions for first medical responders (2005) 🖳 www.resus.org.uk

Anticoagulation

SIGN Antithrombotic therapy (1999) 🖳 www.sign.ac.uk

British Journal of Haematology Guidelines on oral anticoagulation (3rd edition – 1999) **101**: 374–87 🖳 www.bcshguidelines.com

Asthma

British Thoracic Society/SIGN British guideline on the management of asthma (revised 2004) 🖳 www.sign.ac.uk

Peak flow 🖳 www.peakflow.com

British Thoracic Society 🖳 www.brit-thoracic.org.uk
- Current best practice for nebuliser treatment *Thorax* (1997) **52** (Suppl 2): S4–24
- Spirometry in practice: a practical guide to using spirometry in primary care

Cochrane: Accessed via 🖳 www.nelh.nhs.uk
- Abramson *et al.* Allergen immunotherapy for asthma (2003)
- Bhogal *et al.* Written action plans for asthma in children (2005)
- Dennis & Cates Alexander technique for chronic asthma (2000)
- Gibson *et al.* Self-management education and regular practitioner review for adults with asthma (2002)
- Gøtzsche *et al.* House dust mite control measures for asthma (2004)
- Holloway & Ram Breathing exercises for asthma (2004)
- Hondras *et al.* Manual therapy for asthma (2005)
- Kilburn *et al.* Pet allergen control measures for allergic asthma in children and adults (2001)
- McCarney *et al.* Acupuncture for chronic asthma (2003)
- McCarney *et al.* Homeopathy for chronic asthma (2004)
- Ram *et al.* Physical training for asthma (2005)
- Thien *et al.* Dietary marine fatty acids (fish oil) for asthma (2002)
- York & Shuldham Family therapy for chronic asthma in children (2005)

Thorax

- Huntl4ey & Ernst Herbal medicines for asthma: a systematic review (2000) **55**(11): 925–9
- Huntley *et al.* Relaxation therapies for asthma: a systematic review (2002) **57**(2): 127–31

Clinical evidence: Accessed via 🖥 www.nelh.nhs.uk

- Dennis *et al.* Asthma (2004)
- Keeley & McKean Asthma and other wheezing disorders in children (2004)

BMJ Learning Childhood asthma: diagnosis and treatment 🖥 www.bmjlearning.com

Chronic illness

BMJ Von Korff *et al.* Organizing care for chronic illness (2002) **325**: 92–4 🖥 www.bmj.com

Expert Patient Scheme 🖥 www.expertpatients.nhs.uk

Chronic obstructive pulmonary disease (COPD)

RCP/NICE National clinical guideline on management of chronic obstructive pulmonary disease in adults in primary and secondary care *Thorax* (2004) **59**(Suppl 1): 1–232 🖥 www.nice.org.uk

British Thoracic Society 🖥 www.brit-thoracic.org.uk

- Current best practice for nebuliser treatment *Thorax* (1997) **52**(Suppl 2): S4–24
- Spirometry in practice: a practical guide to using spirometry in primary care

ARTP/BTS Certificate in spirometry – further details and list of approved training centres are available from ☎ 0121 697 8339

Cochrane: Accessed via 🖥 www.nelh.nhs.uk

- Barr *et al.* Tiotropium for stable chronic obstructive pulmonary disease (2005)
- Bradley & O'Neill Short-term ambulatory oxygen for chronic obstructive pulmonary disease (2005)
- Cranston *et al.* Domiciliary oxygen for chronic obstructive pulmonary disease (2005)
- Lacasse *et al.* Pulmonary rehabilitation for chronic obstructive pulmonary disease (2001)
- Turnock *et al.* Action plans for chronic obstructive pulmonary disease (2005)
- Walters *et al.* Oral corticosteroids for stable chronic obstructive pulmonary disease (2005)
- Wood-Baker *et al.* Systemic corticosteroids for acute exacerbations of chronic obstructive pulmonary disease (2005)

Clotting tendencies – see thrombophilia

Cystic fibrosis

CF Trust Standards for the clinical care of children and adults with CF in the UK (2001) ▣ www.cftrust.org.uk

UK Newborn Screening Programme Centre CF screening programme and leaflets about CF screening for parents ▣ www.newbornscreening-bloodspot.org.uk

Diffuse parenchymal lung disease

British Thoracic Society The diagnosis, assessment and treatment of diffuse parenchymal lung disease in adults *Thorax* (1999) **54**(Suppl 1) ▣ www.brit-thoracic.org.uk

Disability and benefits

Department of Work and Pensions (DWP) ▣ www.dwp.gov.uk

DWP *Medical Evidence for Statutory Sick Pay, Statutory Maternity Pay and Social Security Incapacity Benefit Purposes: a guide for registered Medical Practitioners.* IB204. April 2000
▣ www.dwp.gov.uk/medical/medicalib204/index.asp

Disability Discrimination Act ▣ www.disability.gov.uk

Jobcentre Plus ▣ www.jobcentreplus.gov.uk

Diving

British Thoracic Society Guidelines on respiratory aspects of fitness for diving *Thorax* (2003) **58**: 3–13 ▣ www.brit-thoracic.org.uk

Driving

DVLA At-a-glance guide to the current medical standards of fitness to drive for medical practitioners. Available from ▣ www.dvla.gov.uk

Medical advisers from the DVLA can advise on difficult issues – contact: Drivers Medical Unit, DVLA, Swansea SA99 1TU or ☎ 01792 761119

Drugs

BNF ▣ www.bnf.org

Children's BNF ▣ www.bnfc.nhs.uk

Medicines and Healthcare Products Regulatory Agency (MHRA – formerly MCA) ▣ www.mhra.gov.uk

Obtaining steroid cards:
- England and Wales: Department of Health ☎ 08701 555 455
- Scotland: Banner Business Supplies ☎ 01506 448 440

Flying

British Thoracic Society Managing patients with respiratory disease planning air travel *Thorax* (2002) **57**: 289–304

GP contract

DoH The GMS Contract 🖥 www.dh.gov.uk

BMA The Blue Book and supporting documents 🖥 www.bma.org.uk

NHS Employers 🖥 www.nhsemployers.org/primary/index

Hayfever – see rhinitis

Infection (see also pneumonia, influenza and tuberculosis)

Health Protection Agency (HPA) Topics A–Z 🖥 www.hpa.org.uk

RCOG Chickenpox in pregnancy (2001) 🖥 www.rcog.org.uk

DTB Chickenpox, pregnancy and the newborn (2005) **45**(9): 69–72

Hyposplenism/asplenism: patient cards and information sheets are available from: Department of Health, PO Box 410, Wetherby, LS23 7LL

Influenza

NICE Guidance on the use of zanamivir, oseltamivir and amantadine for the treatment of influenza (2003) 🖥 www.nice.org.uk

Health Protection Agency (HPA) Topics A–Z: Influenza 🖥 www.hpa.org.uk

Doh (Chief Medical Officer) Explaining pandemic flu (2005) Available from 🖥 www.dh.gov.uk

Lung cancer

SIGN Management of lung cancer (1998) 🖥 www.sign.ac.uk

Occupational lung disease

RIDDOR incident contact centre ☎ 0845 300 99 23 🖥 www.riddor.gov.uk

Health and Safety Executive ☎ 0870 154 55 00 🖥 www.hse.gov.uk

Jobcentre Plus 🖥 www.jobcentreplus.gov.uk

Occupational and Environmental Diseases Association 🖥 www.oeda.demon.co.uk

Palliative care

Hospice information ☎ 0870 903 3903
🖳 www.hospiceinformation.info

Woodruff and Doyle *The IAHPC Manual of Palliative Care* (2nd edn)
(2004) IAHPC Press ISBN 0-9758525-1-5
🖳 www.hospicecare.com/manual/toc-main.html

Davis C ABC of palliative care: breathlessness, cough and other respiratory problems *BMJ* (1997) **315**: 931–4 🖳 www.bmj.com

Doyle *et al.* Oxford Textbook of Palliative Medicine (2005) Oxford
University Press ISBN: 0198566980

Watson *et al.* *Oxford Handbook of Palliative Care* (2005) Oxford
University Press ISBN: 0198508972

Pleural effusion

British Thoracic Society Guidelines for the management of pleural
effusion (2003) 🖳 www.brit-thoracic.org.uk

Pneumonia

British Thoracic Society 🖳 www.brit-thoracic.org.uk
- Guidelines for the management of community-acquired pneumonia in
  adults (2001) and Update (2004)
- Guidelines for the management of community-acquired pneumonia in
  children (2002)

Pneumothorax

British Thoracic Society Guidelines for the management of spontaneous pneumothorax (2003) 🖳 www.brit-thoracic.org.uk

Pulmonary hypertension

British Heart Foundation Factfile Pulmonary hypertension (1/2003)
🖳 www.bhf.org.uk

Resuscitation

Resuscitation Council (UK) 🖳 www.resus.org.uk
- Resuscitation guidelines (2000)
- Cardiopulmonary resuscitation guidance for clinical practice and
  training in primary care (2001)
- The use of biphasic defibrillators and AEDs in children (revised 2003)

BMA, Royal College of Nursing and Resuscitation Council (UK)
Decisions relating to cardiopulmonary resuscitation (2001)
🖳 www.resus.org.uk

Rhinitis

British Society for Allergy and Clinical Immunology (BSACI) Rhinitis
management guidelines (2000) 🖳 www.bsaci.org

Sleep apnoea

SIGN/British Thoracic Society Management of obstructive sleep apnoea/hypopnoea syndrome in adults (2003) 🖳 www.sign.ac.uk

Smoking

Clinical Evidence: Thorogood *et al.* Cardiovascular disorders: changing behaviour (2003) Accessed via 🖳 www.nelh.nhs.uk

NICE 🖳 www.nice.org.uk
- Smoking cessation: brief interventions and referral for smoking cessation in primary care and other settings (2006)
- Nicotine replacement and bupropion for smoking cessation (2002)

Cochrane: Accessed via 🖳 www.nelh.nhs.uk
- Abbot *et al.* Hypnotherapy for smoking cessation (1998)
- Hughes *et al.* Antidepressants for smoking cessation (2004)
- Silagy *et al.* Nicotine replacement for smoking cessation (2004)
- Stead & Lancaster Group behaviour therapy programmes for smoking cessation (2005)

Thorax Smoking cessation guidelines for health professionals: an update (2000) **55**: 987–90 🖳 http://thorax.bmjjournals.com

Russell MAH Effect of GPs' advice against smoking *BMJ* (1979) **2**: 231–5

Thrombophilia

British Committee for Standards in Haematology Diagnosis and management of heritable thrombophilia (2001) 🖳 www.bcshguidelines.com

Thrombosis/thromboembolic disease

RCOG 🖳 www.rcog.org.uk
- Thromboprophylaxis during pregnancy, labour and after vaginal delivery (2004)
- Thromboembolic disease in pregnancy and the puerperium (2001)

SIGN Antithrombotic therapy (1999) 🖳 www.sign.ac.uk

British Journal of Haematology Guidelines on oral anticoagulation (3rd edition – 1999) **101**: 374–87 🖳 www.bcshguidelines.com

Tuberculosis

British Thoracic Society 🖳 www.brit-thoracic.org.uk
- Chemotherapy and management of tuberculosis in the UK *Thorax* (1998) **53**(7): 536–48
- Control and prevention of tuberculosis in the UK: code of practice *Thorax* (2000) **55**: 887–901

Health Protection Agency (HPA) Topics A–Z: Tuberculosis 🖳 www.hpa.org.uk

DoH Stopping tuberculosis in England: an action plan from the Chief Medical Officer (2004) 🖳 www.dh.gov.uk

Information and contacts for patients, relatives and carers

General information

British Lung Foundation ☎ 08458 50 50 20 🖳 www.lunguk.org

DIPEx patient experience database 🖳 www.dipex.org

Expert Patient Scheme 🖳 www.expertpatients.nhs.uk

Patient UK Patient information on a range of topics
🖳 www.patient.co.uk

ENT UK 🖳 www.entuk.org

National Electronic Library for Health 🖳 www.nelh.nhs.uk

Allergy/anaphylaxis

Allergy UK ☎ 01322 619898 🖳 www.allergyuk.org

Anaphylaxis Campaign ☎ 01252 542029 🖳 www.anaphylaxis.org.uk

Medic-Alert Foundation: supply Medic-Alert bracelets
☎ 0800 581 420 🖳 www.medicalert.co.uk

Asthma

Asthma UK ☎ 08457 01 02 03 🖳 www.asthma.org.uk

Benefits

Benefit fraud line ☎ 0800 85 44 40

Citizens' Advice Bureau 🖳 www.adviceguide.org.uk

Department of Work and Pensions 🖳 www.dwp.gov.uk ☎ *Benefits enquiry line* 0800 882200; 0800 243355 (minicom facility); 0800 441144 (for help with form completion)

Government information and services 🖳 www.direct.gov.uk

HM Revenue and Customs 🖳 www.hmrc.gov.uk *Tax credit enquiry line* ☎ 0845 300 3900

Jobcentre Plus 🖳 www.jobcentreplus.gov.uk

Pension Service 🖳 www.thepensionservice.gov.uk

Veterans Agency ☎ 0800 169 22 77 🖳 www.veteransagency.mod.uk

Carers

Carers UK ☎ 0808 808 7777 🖳 www.carersonline.org.uk

Counsel and Care ☎ 0845 300 7585 🖳 www.counselandcare.org.uk

Princess Royal Trust for Carers ☎ 020 7480 7788 🖳 www.carers.org

Disability and carers' service 🖳 www.disability.gov.uk

Cystic fibrosis

Cystic Fibrosis Trust 🖳 www.cftrust.org.uk

UK Newborn Screening Programme Centre Leaflets about CF screening for parents 🖳 www.newbornscreening-bloodspot.org.uk

Disability

Disabled Living Foundation ☎ 0845 130 9177 🖳 www.dlf.org.uk

Citizens' Advice Bureau 🖳 www.adviceguide.org.uk

Royal Association for Disability and Rehabilitation (RADAR) ☎ 020 7250 3222 🖳 www.radar.org.uk

Disablement Information and Advice Line (DIAL) ☎ 01302 310123 🖳 www.dialuk.info

Mobility Advice and Vehicle Information Service (MAVIS) 🖳 www.dft.gov.uk/access/mavis

Motability 🖳 www.motability.co.uk

Elderly

Age Concern ☎ 0800 00 99 66 🖳 www.ageconcern.org.uk

Help the Aged ☎ 0800 800 65 65 🖳 www.helptheaged.org.uk

Immunization

Immunization NHS website for patients 🖳 www.immunisation.org.uk

Infection

Health Protection Agency (HPA) Topics A–Z: TB and BCG 🖳 www.hpa.org.uk

The Aspergillus Website 🖳 www.aspergillus.man.ac.uk

Lung cancer

Lung cancer resources directory 🖳 www.cancerindex.org

The Roy Castle Lung Cancer Foundation ☎ 0800 358 7200 🖳 www.roycastle.org

Cancerbacup ☎ 0808 800 1234 🖳 www.cancerbacup.org.uk

Macmillan Cancer Relief ☎ 0808 808 2020 🖳 www.macmillan.org.uk

Occupational lung disease

Occupational and Environmental Diseases Association
🖳 www.oeda.demon.co.uk

Sleep apnoea

The Sleep Apnoea Trust (SATA) ☎ 01494 527772
🖳 www.sleep-apnoea-trust.org

Smoking

Action on Smoking and Health (ASH) ☎ 020 7739 5902
🖳 www.ash.org.uk

NHS smoking helpline ☎ 0800 169 0 169; pregnancy smoking helpline
☎ 0800 169 9 169 🖳 www.givingupsmoking.co.uk

Quit helpline ☎ 0800 00 22 00 🖳 www.quit.org.uk

Thrombosis

Lifeblood: the thrombosis charity ☎ 01406 381017
🖳 www.thrombosis-charity.org.uk

Appendix

Acute treatment algorithms

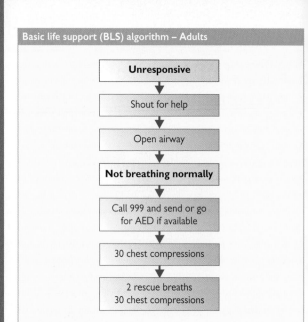

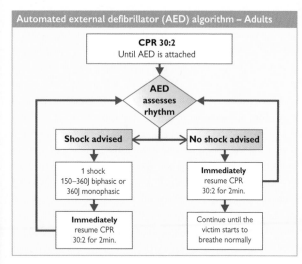

262

The BLS and AED algorithms are reproduced from the Resuscitation guidelines (2005) with permission ▣ www.resus.org.uk

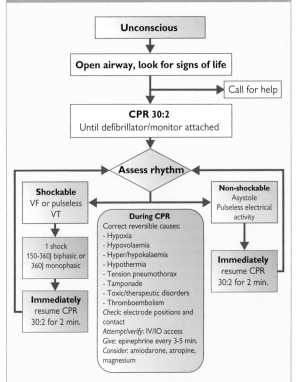

Unconscious

Open airway, look for signs of life

Call for help

CPR 30:2
Until defibrillator/monitor attached

Assess rhythm

Shockable
VF or pulseless VT

Non-shockable
Asystole
Pulseless electrical activity

1 shock
150-360J biphasic or 360J monophasic

During CPR
Correct reversible causes:
- Hypoxia
- Hypovolaemia
- Hyper/hypokalaemia
- Hypothermia
- Tension pneumothorax
- Tamponade
- Toxic/therapeutic disorders
- Thromboembolism
Check: electrode positions and contact
Attempt/verify: IV/IO access
Give: epinephrine every 3-5 min.
Consider: amiodarone, atropine, magnesium

Immediately
resume CPR 30:2 for 2 min.

Immediately
resume CPR 30:2 for 2 min.

Pad position: Place 1 pad to the right of the sternum below the clavicile. Place the order pad vertically in the midaxillary line approximately level with the V6 ECG electrode position or female breast (though clear of any breast tissue).

⚠ Give adrenaline 1mg IV immediately before alternate shocks, i.e. ≈ every 3–5min.

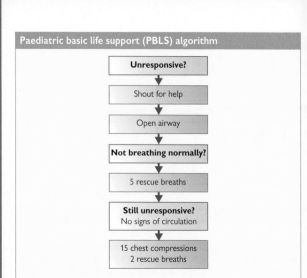

Paediatric basic life support (PBLS) algorithm

Unresponsive?

↓

Shout for help

↓

Open airway

↓

Not breathing normally?

↓

5 rescue breaths

↓

Still unresponsive?
No signs of circulation

↓

15 chest compressions
2 rescue breaths

After 1 minute call for help then continue CPR

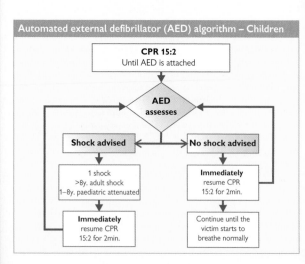

Automated external defibrillator (AED) algorithm – Children

CPR 15:2
Until AED is attached

↓

AED assesses

Shock advised ←→ **No shock advised**

1 shock
>8y. adult shock
1–8y. paediatric attenuated

Immediately resume CPR 15:2 for 2min.

Immediately resume CPR 15:2 for 2min.

Continue until the victim starts to breathe normally

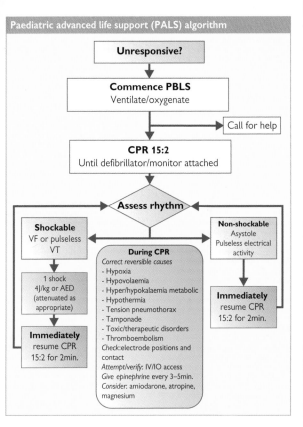

Unresponsive?

Commence PBLS
Ventilate/oxygenate

Call for help

CPR 15:2
Until defibrillator/monitor attached

Assess rhythm

Shockable
VF or pulseless VT

1 shock
4J/kg or AED
(attenuated as appropriate)

Immediately
resume CPR
15:2 for 2min.

During CPR
Correct reversible causes
- Hypoxia
- Hypovolaemia
- Hyper/hypokalaemia metabolic
- Hypothermia
- Tension pneumothorax
- Tamponade
- Toxic/therapeutic disorders
- Thromboembolism
Check: electrode positions and contact
Attempt/verify: IV/IO access
Give epinephrine every 3–5min.
Consider: amiodarone, atropine, magnesium

Non-shockable
Asystole
Pulseless electrical activity

Immediately
resume CPR
15:2 for 2min.

Adrenaline (epinephrine) dose

- Intravenous or interosseous (IO) access – 10mcgm/kg epinephrine (0.1ml/kg of 1:10,000 solution).
- If circulatory access is not present, and can't be quickly obtained, but the child has a tracheal tube in place, consider giving adrenaline 100mcgm/kg via the tracheal tube (1ml/kg of 1:10,000 or 0.1ml/kg of 1:1,000 solution). This is the least satisfactory route of administration.

⚠ Don't give 1:1000 epinephrine IV or IO.

⚠ If blockage of the airway is only partial, the victim will usually be able to dislodge the foreign body by coughing. If obstruction is complete, urgent intervention is required to prevent asphyxia.

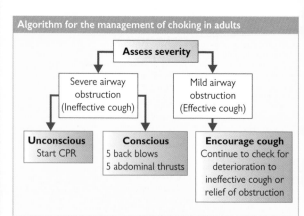

Algorithm for the management of choking in adults

Assess severity

Severe airway obstruction (Ineffective cough)

Mild airway obstruction (Effective cough)

Unconscious
Start CPR

Conscious
5 back blows
5 abdominal thrusts

Encourage cough
Continue to check for deterioration to ineffective cough or relief of obstruction

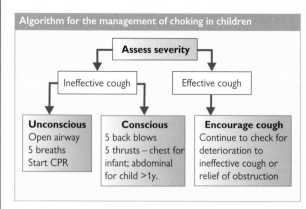

Algorithm for the management of choking in children

Assess severity

Ineffective cough

Effective cough

Unconscious
Open airway
5 breaths
Start CPR

Conscious
5 back blows
5 thrusts – chest for infant; abdominal for child >1y.

Encourage cough
Continue to check for deterioration to ineffective cough or relief of obstruction

266

⚠ Do not perform blind finger sweeps of the mouth or upper airway as these may further impact a foreign body or cause soft tissue damage

Algorithms are reproduced with permission from the Resuscitation Council (UK)
🖳 www.resus.org.uk

Anaphylactic reactions: treatment algorithm for adults and children

Consider anaphylaxis when compatible history of severe allergic-type reaction with respiratory difficulty and/or hypotension especially if skin changes present

↓

Give oxygen treatment when available

↓

Stridor, wheeze, respiratory distress or clinical signs of shock

↓

Adrenaline (epinephrine) 1:1000 solution
>12y.: 0.5ml (500 micrograms) IM – 0.25ml (250 micrograms) if the child is small or pre-pubertal
6–12y.: 0.25ml (250 micrograms) IM
>6mo.–6y: 0.12ml (120 micrograms) IM
<6mo.: 0.05ml (50 micrograms) IM

↓

Repeat in 5 minutes if no clinical improvement

↓

Antihistamine (chlorphenamine)
>12y.: 10–20mg IM
6–12y.: 5–10mg IM
1–6y.: 2.5–5mg IM

↓

In addition

For all severe or recurrent reactions and patients with asthma give hydrocortisone
>12.: 100–500mg IM or slow IV
6–12y.: 100mg IM or slow IV
1–6.: 50mg IM or slow IV

If clinical manifestations of shock do not respond to drug treatment give 20ml/kg of IV fluids if available (1–2l for an adult). Rapid infusion or one repeat dose may be needed

267

Management of acute severe asthma in adults in general practice

Moderate asthma	Acute severe asthma	Life-threatening asthma
Initial assessment		
PEFR >50% best or predicted	PEFR 33–50% best or predicted	PEFR <33% best or predicted
Further assessment		
Speech normal Respiration <25 breaths/min. Pulse <110 beats/min.	Can't complete sentences Respiration ≥25 breaths/min. Pulse ≥ 110 beats/min.	Oxygen saturation <92% Silent chest, cyanosis or feeble respiratory effort Bradycardia, dysrhythmia or hypotension Exhaustion, confusion or coma
Management		
Treat at home or in the surgery and ASSESS RESPONSE TO TREATMENT	Consider admission	Arrange immediate admission
Treatment		
High dose β₂ bronchodilator. Ideally via oxygen-driven nebulizer (salbutamol 5mg or terbutaline 10mg). Alternatively use air-driven nebulizer or inhaler via spacer (1 puff 10–20x) *If PEFR >50–75% predicted/best:* Give prednisolone 40–50mg Continue or step up usual treatment *If good response to first nebulized treatment* (symptoms improved, respiration and pulse settling and PEFR >50%) continue or step up usual treatment and continue prednisolone	*Oxygen 40–60% if available* *High dose β₂ bronchodilator.* Ideally via oxygen-driven nebulizer (salbutamol 5mg or terbutaline 10mg). Alternatively use air-driven nebulizer or inhaler via spacer (1 puff 10–20x) *Prednisolone 40–50mg or IV hydrocortisone 100mg* *If no response in acute, severe asthma:* ADMIT	*Oxygen 40–60% if available* *Prednisolone 40–50mg or IV hydrocortisone 100mg immediately* *High dose β₂ bronchodilator.* Ideally via oxygen-driven nebulizer (salbutamol 5mg or terbutaline 10mg). Alternatively use air-driven nebulizer or inhaler via spacer (1 puff 10–20x) *ADMIT immediately*

ASSESS ASTHMA SEVERITY		
Moderate exacerbation	Severe exacerbation	Life-threatening asthma
Oxygen saturation ≥92% PEFR ≥50% best or predicted Able to talk Heart rate ≤120/min. Respiratory rate ≤30/min.	Oxygen saturation <92% PEFR <50% best or predicted Too breathless to talk Heart rate >120/min. Respiratory rate >30/min. Use of accessory neck muscles	Oxygen saturation <92% PEFR <33% best or predicted Silent chest Poor respiratory effort Agitation Altered consciousness Cyanosis
β₂ agonist 2–4 puffs via spacer Consider soluble prednisolone 30–40mg **Increase β₂ agonist dose by 2 puffs every 2min. up to 10 puffs according to response**	Oxygen via face mask β₂ agonist 10 puffs via spacer ± facemask or nebulized salbutamol 2.5–5mg (or terbutaline 5–10mg) Soluble prednisolone 30–40mg **Assess response to treatment 15min. after β₂ agonist**	Oxygen via face mask Nebulize: -salbutamol 5mg or terbutaline 10mg + -ipratropium 0.25mg Soluble prednisolone 30–40mg or IV hydrocortisone 100mg
IF POOR RESPONSE ARRANGE ADMISSION	IF POOR RESPONSE REPEAT β₂ AGONIST AND ARRANGE ADMISSION	REPEAT β₂ AGONIST VIA OXYGEN-DRIVEN NEBULIZER WHILST ARRANGING IMMEDIATE HOSPITAL ADMISSION

GOOD RESPONSE	POOR RESPONSE
Continue up to 10 puffs or nebulized β2 agonist as needed (max. every 4h.) **If symptoms are not controlled repeat β₂ agonist and refer to hospital** Continue prednisolone for up to 3d. Arrange follow-up clinic visit	Stay with the patient until the ambulance arrives Send written assessment and referral details Repeat β₂ agonist via oxygen-driven nebulizer in the ambulance

269

⚠ *Lower threshold for admission if*

• Attack in late afternoon or at night
• Recent hospital admission or previous severe attack
• Concern over social circumstances or ability to cope at home

Algorithm reproduced from the British guideline on the management of asthma (2004) with permission from SIGN/British Thoracic Society.

Management of acute asthma in children 2–5y. in general practice

ASSESS ASTHMA SEVERITY		
Moderate exacerbation	Severe exacerbation	Life-threatening asthma
Oxygen saturation ≥92% Able to talk Heart rate ≤130/min. Respiratory rate ≤50/min.	Oxygen saturation <92% Too breathless to talk Heart rate >130/min. Respiratory rate >50/min. Use of accessory neck muscles	Oxygen saturation <92% Silent chest Poor respiratory effort Agitation Altered consciousness Cyanosis
β_2 agonist 2–4 puffs via spacer Consider soluble prednisolone 20mg **Increase β_2 agonist dose by 2 puffs every 2min. up to 10 puffs according to response**	Oxygen via face mask β_2 agonist 10 puffs via spacer ± facemask or nebulized salbutamol 2.5–5mg (or terbutaline 5mg) Soluble prednisolone 20mg **Assess response to treatment 15min. after β_2 agonist**	Oxygen via face mask Nebulize: -salbutamol 2.5mg or terbutaline 5mg + -ipratropium 0.25mg Soluble prednisolone 20mg or IV hydrocortisone 50mg
IF POOR RESPONSE ARRANGE ADMISSION	IF POOR RESPONSE REPEAT β_2 AGONIST AND ARRANGE ADMISSION	REPEAT β_2 AGONIST VIA OXYGEN-DRIVEN NEBULIZER WHILST ARRANGING IMMEDIATE HOSPITAL ADMISSION

GOOD RESPONSE	POOR RESPONSE
Continue up to 10 puffs or nebulized β2 agonist as needed (max. every 4h.) **If symptoms are not controlled repeat β_2 agonist and refer to hospital** Continue prednisolone for up to 3d. Arrange follow-up clinic visit	Stay with the patient until the ambulance arrives Send written assessment and referral details Repeat β_2 agonist via oxygen-driven nebulizer in the ambulance

⚠ *Lower threshold for admission if*
• Attack in late afternoon or at night
• Recent hospital admission or previous severe attack
• Concern over social circumstances or ability to cope at home

Algorithm reproduced from the British guideline on the management of asthma (2004) with permission from SIGN/British Thoracic Society.

Index

271